D0268989

A Nurse's Guide to Caring for Cardiac Intervention Patients

A Nurse's Guide to Caring for Cardiac Intervention Patients

By

EILEEN O'GRADY RN BSc

Interventional Cardiology Unit, Leeds General Infirmary

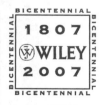

John Wiley & Sons, Ltd

Telephone (+44) 1243 779777

Email (for orders and customer service enquiries): cs-books@wiley.co.uk
Visit our Home Page on www.wileyeurope.com or www.wiley.com

Other Wiley Editorial Offices

John Wiley & Sons Inc., 111 River Street, Hoboken, NJ 07030, USA

Jossey-Bass, 989 Market Street, San Francisco, CA 94103-1741, USA

Wiley-VCH Verlag GmbH, Boschstr. 12, D-69469 Weinheim, Germany

John Wiley & Sons Australia Ltd, 42 McDougall Street, Milton, Queensland 4064, Australia

John Wiley & Sons (Asia) Pte Ltd, 2 Clementi Loop #02-01, Jin Xing Distripark, Singapore 129809

John Wiley & Sons Canada Ltd, 6045 Freemont Blvd, Mississauga, Ontario, L5R 4J3, Canada

Wiley also publishes its books in a variety of electronic formats. Some content that appears in print may not be available in electronic books.

Anniversary Logo Design: Richard J. Pacifico

Library of Congress Cataloging-in-Publication Data:

O'Grady, Eileen.
A Nurse's Guide to Caring for Cardiac Intervention Patients / Eileen O'Grady.
p. ; cm.
Includes bibliographical references.
ISBN-13: 978-0-470-01995-5 (alk. paper)
ISBN-10: 0-470-01995-6 (alk. paper)
1. Heart – Diseases – Nursing. 2. Heart – Diseases – Patients – Rehabilitation. 3. Coronary heart disease. I. Title.
[DNLM: 1. Heart Diseases – nursing. WY 152.5 O35c 2007]
RC674.O327 2007
616.1'20231 – dc22

2006022726

British Library Cataloguing in Publication Data

A catalogue record for this book is available from the British Library

ISBN-13: 978-0-470-01995-5

Typeset in 10/12pt Times by Laserwords Private Limited, Chennai, India
Printed and bound in Great Britain by TJ International, Padstow, Cornwall
This book is printed on acid-free paper responsibly manufactured from sustainable forestry in which at least two trees are planted for each one used for paper production.

Contents

Preface

Since the publication of the *National Service Framework for Coronary Heart Disease* (NSFCHD), in March 2000, the number of interventional cardiac procedures being performed in England has grown and continues to grow. In order to achieve the NSFCHD targets, more district general hospitals (DGHs) are now performing procedures previously only carried out in tertiary centres, such as electrophysiology and ablation, as well as routine, low-risk percutaneous coronary intervention (PCI) and implantable cardioverter defibrillator (ICD) implantation.

The role of the cardiac nurse in the DGH will evolve to provide efficient and effective care for these patients. As a staff nurse working in Leeds General Infirmary – one of the busiest cardiology interventional centres in England – I found it difficult to find a book explaining various procedures from a nursing perspective. Therefore, using experience gained on the ward, latest research studies and evidence-based practice, this book aims to:

- outline how to care for such patients pre and post procedure;
- provide guidance for when speaking to patients and their families;
- help to recognise and deal with potential complications.

Cardiology is research-driven; therefore protocols vary from hospital to hospital and change in accordance with the latest research findings and cardiologist preference. This book aims to guide nurses through interventional cardiology even though local protocols may differ from what is suggested in the book.

The glossary can be found at the back of the book. This serves not only to explain terms used throughout the book, but can also be used as a quick reference guide and is eminently readable and informative as a stand-alone chapter.

ACKNOWLEDGEMENTS

I would like to thank all of my colleagues at Leeds General Infirmary for their patience and support, especially those who took the time to read a chapter and provided valuable feedback, suggestions and alterations.

All illustrations have been created by Steve Granshaw. I would like to thank Steve for his superb artwork and knowledge on how to use a computer.

DISCLAIMER

upon as recommending or promoting a specific method, diagnosis, or treatment by nurses and healthcare workers for any particular patient. The publisher and the author make no representations or warranties with respect to the accuracy or completeness of the contents of this work and specifically disclaim all warranties, including without limitation any implied warranties of fitness for a particular purpose. In view of ongoing research, equipment modifications, changes in governmental regulations, and the constant flow of information relating to the use of medicines, equipment, and devices, the reader is urged to review and evaluate the information provided in the package insert or instructions for each medicine, equipment, or device for, among other things, any changes in the instructions or indication of usage and for added warnings and precautions. Readers should consult with a specialist where appropriate. The fact that an organization or Website is referred to in this work as a citation and/or a potential source of further information does not mean that the author or the publisher endorses the information the organization or Website may provide or recommendations it may make. Further, readers should be aware that Internet Websites listed in this work may have changed or disappeared between when this work was written and when it is read. No warranty may be created or extended by any promotional statements for this work. Neither the publisher nor the author shall be liable for any damages arising herefrom.

1 Access Sites of Percutaneous Procedures

In 1929, Werner Forssman performed the first human cardiac catheterisation by passing a urethral catheter from his left antecubital vein into the right side of his heart (10). Cardiac catheterisation has evolved since then and nowadays is used in a variety of procedures that vary from investigative tests such as angiograms to interventions such as coronary angioplasty and atrial septal defect repairs, thus reducing the need for cardiac surgery (11).

These can be referred to as percutaneous coronary procedures, as the heart is accessed by inserting a catheter through the skin into an artery and/or vein, and threading it up to the heart. Access to the arterial system may be via the femoral, brachial or radial artery (5).

ADVANTAGES OF PERCUTANEOUS ACCESS

The majority of percutaneous coronary investigations and interventions are performed under local anaesthetic, as patients may be asked to cough, hold their breath or move their position during the procedure. Using a local anaesthetic also has the advantage of avoiding the risks associated with general anaesthesia (11). The other advantages that percutaneous coronary procedures offer over cardiac surgery include:

- Patients are less anxious waiting for a percutaneous procedure than for a surgical procedure (8).
- A cardiopulmonary bypass machine, if required, and its inherent risks are avoided (8).
- The hospital stay is shorter. For example, patients undergoing percutaneous coronary intervention (PCI) normally stay in hospital for 12–24 hours, whereas patients undergoing a coronary artery bypass graft (CABG) require a stay of 3–7 days (8).
- Barring complications, the average cost of percutaneous coronary procedures is substantially lower than that of surgery (8).
- Patients are able to resume their normal life sooner after percutaneous procedures. For example, patients can usually return to work within 7–10 days after a PCI, whereas patients undergoing a CABG return to work within 6 weeks (8).

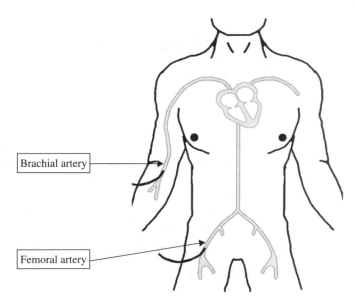

Figure 1.1. Introducing a catheter into the brachial or femoral artery.

• If a patient has a clotting disorder or has recently had thrombolysis, they can be treated in an emergency with PCI (1).

SELECTING THE ARTERIAL PUNCTURE

The access site is selected by the cardiologist prior to the procedure; however, the femoral artery is the preferred access site to the arterial system for the majority of percutaneous procedures (see Figure 1.1). Although the brachial and radial arteries may be preferred by some cardiologists, they are mainly used if the femoral artery is unavailable, due to peripheral vascular disease, for example, or if the patient is unable to lie flat on their back during the procedure, such as patients with severe heart failure, who would normally sleep with three or four pillows (9).

The brachial and radial arteries are smaller than the femoral artery and carry a higher risk of dissection and occlusion. Percutaneous puncture of the brachial artery is more likely to require surgical repair than percutaneous femoral puncture. In addition to this, brachial arteriotomy under direct vision can be technically challenging for the inexperienced operator and is time-consuming (9).

Percutaneous radial artery puncture appears safe, but it results in occlusion of the radial artery in around 5% of cases. Although, in such cases, the blood to the hand would be supplied by the ulnar artery, the occluded radial artery would not be available for a CABG surgery if the patient required one in the future (9).

FEMORAL ACCESS

The most common vascular access site is the femoral artery. It can also be referred to as the Judkin's approach (7). The selected femoral artery is shaved of groin hair in order to reduce infection risk and then the area is liberally cleaned with antiseptic solution (8). Then, a local anaesthetic such as lignocaine is slowly injected into the inguinal area of the groin, as a slow injection of the local anaesthetic is less painful for the patient and produces better tissue infiltration (2).

Once the femoral area is anaesthetised, the cardiologist punctures the femoral artery percutaneously by inserting a large cannula containing a removable obturator. The presence of blood flow once the obturator is removed confirms that this cannula is within the lumen of the artery. Once proper placement is established, a guidewire is introduced through the cannula into the artery to the level of the diaphragm. The cannula is then removed and replaced by a valved introducer sheath (known as a femoral sheath) (8). The patient may feel some pushing and tugging at this time. This introducer sheath provides haemostasis and support at the puncture site and reduces potential arterial trauma if multiple catheter exchanges are necessary (8).

The femoral vein is accessed in a similar manner if it is required. Venous access is mainly used during electrophysiological studies (EPS) and radio-frequency ablation (RFA). Venous access for temporary pacing is no longer routine during PCI; however, it should be considered for high-risk patients, such as those with acute myocardial infarction (MI) or left bundle branch block needing right coronary artery PCI, or if a rotoblator or thrombus aspiration device is required (6).

REMOVING A FEMORAL SHEATH

There are several methods of obtaining haemostasis in the femoral puncture site post sheath removal. Closure devices, such as AngioSeal, VasoSeal, Duett and Perclose, allow the removal of the femoral sheath at the end of the procedure, no matter what the anticoagulation status is (9). However, the majority of centres still rely on the compression of the femoral artery using either manual or mechanical compression, or a combination (4). This means that the femoral sheath is usually removed 3–4 hours after the procedure if heparin has been used, such as during PCI (8). As femoral sheaths are usually removed on the ward by nursing staff, it is discussed in more detail in Chapter 2.

RADIAL ACCESS

The radial artery approach was developed as an alternative to the percutaneous transbrachial approach in an attempt to limit vascular complications. The inherent advantages of the transradial approach are that the hand has a dual arterial supply

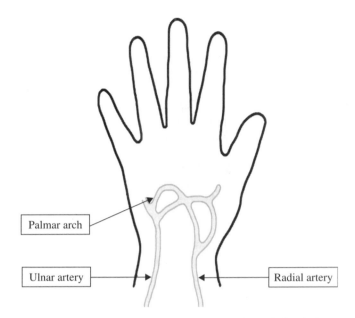

Figure 1.2. Radial artery anatomy and collateral circulation.

connected via the palmar arches and that there are no nerves or veins at the site of puncture (3). The location of the radial artery enables easy access in most people, and it is easier to control bleeding (see Figure 1.2). In addition, prolonged bed rest is unnecessary after the procedure (6).

Although using the radial approach is associated with fewer severe access site-related bleeding complications than the femoral approach, the sheath sizes are smaller. They are usually limited to size 6 or 7 French, and therefore would not be suitable for cases in which larger catheters are required, such as valvuloplasty or rotablation (7). Unfortunately, the radial artery has a propensity to develop spasm, which may make catheter movement difficult or impossible. This can be overcome by the use of vasodilators and long introducer sheaths when appropriate (6). In addition, radial access is only suitable for left-sided heart catheterisation; another approach would be required if the right side of the heart required catheterisation as well (3).

Prior to a radial procedure, the clinician must complete an Allen's test to assess the ulnar artery in the arm to be proceeded on. First, the radial and ulnar arteries are occluded simultaneously while the patient makes a fist. Then, when the hand is opened, it appears blanched. The ulnar artery is released and the hand colour should return within 8–10 seconds. Satisfactory ulnar flow can also be documented by pulse oximetry (6).

In order to insert the catheter into the radial artery, the selected arm is abducted at a 70° angle on an arm board, and the wrist hyperextended over a gauze roll. It is cleaned liberally with antiseptic. A topical anaesthetic is applied first, as it reduces the amount of lignocaine needed for local infiltration over the radial pulse. Large amounts of lignocaine may obscure the pulse and make cannulation more difficult (6). A small incision is made and an 18-gauge needle is introduced at a 45° angle into the radial artery. A guidewire is inserted first and then a valved introducer sheath. Haemostasis is obtained at the end of the procedure after sheath removal using direct pressure. It is recommended that the arterial puncture site be allowed to bleed for several beats before maintaining direct pressure. The radial pulse should be monitored regularly for several hours after the procedure (3).

SHEATH REMOVAL AND POST-PROCEDURE CARE

Before the sheath is removed, 1 mg of verapamil is given through the sheath to minimise spasm of the radial artery (6).

Although haemostasis can be achieved by applying direct manual pressure over the puncture site, there are several radial haemostat devices available on the market, and their guidelines should be followed. The following is a description of one such device. A plastic bracelet with a pressure pad is placed around the wrist. Gauze is wrapped around the plastic strip to prevent skin injury when the bracelet is tightened. Another folded piece of gauze is placed under the pressure pad over the sheath insertion site. While the operator presses the pad over the puncture site, the sheath is withdrawn gently and the bracelet is tightened. The pad is pressed down and locked over the puncture by tightening of the bracelet bracket. The bracelet should be tight enough to ensure haemostasis but not occlude flow to the hand. The patient is checked 1–2 hours later, and the bracelet is loosened. The patient can be discharged 2 hours later and the bracelet removed at home. The patient should be given instructions about puncture site compression with the fingers if later bleeding occurs (6).

BRACHIAL ACCESS

There are two methods of obtaining brachial access, but they should be reserved for patients in whom the radial artery cannot be used (6).

PERCUTANEOUS BRACHIAL ARTERY PUNCTURE

Percutaneous arterial puncture is a safe and effective alternative to brachial artery cut-down, and is normally favoured over the brachial artery cut-down. Although it is similar to femoral arterial puncture, there are several important differences:

1. The brachial artery is smaller (3–5 mm in diameter) than the femoral artery.
2. Because of relatively loose subcutaneous tissues, the course of the brachial artery may change considerably.
3. Spasm can occur easily, with considerable decrease in pulse amplitude, making the puncture more difficult.

4. The artery is more mobile than the femoral artery.
5. The median nerve lies very close to the artery. Accidental touching of the median nerve causes a peculiar electrical shock sensation in the hand.
6. Care should be taken to puncture the artery on the first attempt. Because of the smaller space in the arm, uncontrolled haematoma formation here can readily cause compression syndrome with ischaemia of the forearm and hand (6).

The brachial artery can accommodate up to size 8 French sheath in large men. However, in most patients, especially smaller men and women, smaller sheaths (less than or equal to 6 French) are preferred (6). The brachial and radial pulses should be checked prior to attempting a brachial puncture. They should be strong and equal in both arms. The patency of the ulnar artery should be checked by the Allen's test (6).

The arterial sheath is removed at the end of the procedure and haemostasis is achieved by applying 15–20 minutes of manual pressure until the bleeding has stopped. The arm circumference at the site of the puncture should be measured to facilitate the detection of haematoma formation. The patient should be instructed to keep the arm in a relaxed position for 4–6 hours. Although the patient is allowed to sit up in bed, ambulation should be restricted until these 4–6 hours are completed, to ensure haemostasis (6).

BRACHIAL CUT-DOWN/SONES PROCEDURE

The brachial cut-down procedure is also known as the Sones procedure. This procedure is rarely performed nowadays, as radial access or brachial puncture is favoured over it. Unlike the other procedures, this is not a percutaneous procedure. Once the brachial area is anaesthetised, the brachial artery is accessed by making an incision close to the crease in the elbow. The selected artery is brought to the surface and is used to insert the appropriate catheters for the procedure. Once the procedure is completed, the artery is sutured to prevent bleeding, and then the incision is sutured. If non-absorbable sutures are used on the incision, they will need to be removed in 7–10 days. The wound should be covered with a firm dressing (2).

There is no need for the patient to be kept flat or motionless following a brachial cut-down procedure. They may sit up, eat and mobilise to the bathroom. If the patient has a strong radial pulse, they can be discharged home after 4–6 hours' observation (2).

REFERENCES

1. Al-Obaidi, M., Noble, M. and Siva, A. (2004) *Crash Course Cardiology*, 2nd edn, London, Mosby.
2. Baim, D. S. (2006) *Grossman's Cardiac Catheterisation: Angiography and Intervention*, 7th edn, Philadelphia, Lippincott Williams & Wilkins.

3. Braunweld, E., Zipes, D. and Libby, P. (2001) *Heart Disease: A Textbook of Cardiovascular Medicine*, Vol. 1, 6th edn, London, W.B. Saunders Co.
4. Galli, G. (2005) 'Ask the experts: Re removing arterial and venous sheaths after PCI', *Critical Care Nurse*, available online at *www.findarticles.com*.
5. Julian, D. G., Cowan, J. C. and McLenachan, J. M. (2005) *Cardiology*, 8th edn, London, Elsevier Saunders.
6. Kern, M. (2003) *The Cardiac Catheterisation Handbook*, 4th edn, London, Mosby.
7. Montalsecot, G., Andersen, H., Antoniucer, D., Betriu, A., de Boer, M., Grip, L., *et al.* (2004) 'Recommendations on percutaneous coronary intervention for the reperfusion of acute ST elevation myocardial infarction', *Heart*, 90, available online at *http://heart.bmjjournals.com/cgi/content/full/90/6/e37*.
8. Morton, P. G., Fontaine, D. K., Hudak, C. M. and Gallo, B. M. (2005) *Critical Care Nursing: A Holistic Approach*, 8th edn, Philadelphia, Lippincott Williams & Wilkins.
9. Norell, M. and Perrins, J. (2003) *Essential Interventional Cardiology*, Philadelphia, PA, W.B. Saunders Co.
10. Rosendorff, C. (2005) *Essential Cardiology: Principles and Practice*, 2nd edn, Totowa, New Jersey, Humana Press.
11. Swanton, R. H. (2003) *Pocket Consultant Cardiology*, 5th edn, Oxford, Blackwell Publishing.

2 Removal of Femoral Sheaths

There are three arterial access approaches commonly used for cardiac catheterisation procedures and interventions: radial, brachial and femoral. Although the radial and the brachial artery allow the majority of patients to mobilise immediately after the procedure, the femoral artery is easier to access and allows larger introducer sheaths to be used (10). Therefore, the majority of patients undergoing cardiac catheterisation procedures and interventions will have an introducer sheath percutaneously introduced into either their left or right femoral artery (11). This is commonly referred to as a femoral sheath. Occasionally, an introducer sheath may be inserted into the femoral vein during the procedure if a temporary pacing wire is required or peripheral venous access was a problem (8).

A large proportion of complications associated with cardiac catheterisation procedures and interventions are associated with the arterial access puncture site (2). These complications include: bleeding at the arterial site; haematoma formation; arterial pseudoaneurysm; arteriovenous fistulae; arterial occlusion; distal ischaemia or necrosis; vasovagal response resulting in hypotension and bradycardia. Therefore, in order to minimise these complications, femoral sheaths should be removed by trained personnel (12).

REMOVING SHEATHS USING ARTERIAL CLOSURE DEVICES

Anticoagulants such as heparin or bivalirudin may be required during cardiac interventions and they are usually allowed to dissipate before the femoral sheath is removed (12). Therefore, the femoral sheath may be removed several hours after the procedure on the ward. Then, the traditional approach is to apply manual pressure to the femoral artery for 10–20 minutes, until haemostasis is achieved. The disadvantages of manual compression are that it is time-consuming and uncomfortable for the operator, as a reasonable degree of force is required (12).

Several devices have been developed so that femoral sheaths can be removed immediately at the end of the procedure, no matter what the anticoagulation status is. There are four arterial closure devices currently available: two collagen plug devices (AngioSeal, VasoSeal), a liquid plug (Duett) and a percutaneous suture closure device (Perclose) (12). Using these devices has not reduced the risks associated with puncture site complications; therefore, the patients should continue to be closely monitored (12). These devices are more comfortable for the patient as pressing on the femoral artery, either manually or with a compression device, can be an uncomfortable experience; these devices reduce the risk of a vasovagal reaction induced by such pressure. As haemostasis is immediate, based on the manufacturers' guidelines, the patients will be able to sit up and mobilise earlier, and therefore could be discharged or transferred earlier (or on the same day) if the patient is stable from a cardiac point of view (2; 17). These devices should be used with caution in patients with peripheral vascular disease or low arterial puncture (8). A downside to the closure devices is the added expense (6).

VASOSEAL

The VasoSeal acts by deploying a collagen plug on the external surface of the artery. The collagen interacts with platelets to create a haemostatic seal directly over the puncture site (2; 12; 17).

ANGIOSEAL

The AngioSeal, like the VasoSeal, uses bovine collagen to seal the arterial puncture site. A flat rectangular plate is deployed inside the artery wall. This acts as an anchor to which a suture carrying a small collagen plug is attached, thus forming a mechanical sandwich around the hole in the artery. The anchor, the suture and the collagen sponge are all fully bio-absorbable (2; 12; 17).

DUETT SEALING DEVICE

A pro-coagulant liquid (a mixture of collagen and fibrin) is placed on the external surface of the artery, thus promoting the body's natural clotting plug at the puncture site. The potential advantages of this device are that no foreign material is left inside the artery and the artery can be re-punctured immediately, if this proves necessary (12).

PERCLOSE DEVICE

Perclose devices enable the cardiologist to suture the arterial puncture hole without direct vision of the artery. Unless some arterial wall damage is present, usually only one or two pairs of sutures around the puncture site are required to close the hole effectively (12; 17).

HINT

Personal experience has found that if the puncture site continues to ooze after using an arterial closure device, manual compression applied for 10–20 minutes may stop the oozing. If this does not work, applying a haemostatic dressing such as Kaltostat over the puncture site and then applying a compression device such as a FemoStop with low pressure for 1–2 hours are usually helpful adjuncts.

Despite the advantages of these devices, many centres rely on compressing the arterial puncture site until the bleeding has stopped, using either manual or mechanical compression, or a combination (6). No matter which type of compression is to be applied, in order to reduce potential complications, the person removing the femoral sheath(s) should address the following problems first.

HAS THE ANTICOAGULANT ADMINISTERED DURING THE PROCEDURE DISSIPATED?

It is recommended practice to administer an anticoagulant during cardiac catheterisation or intervention when the procedure is expected to be longer than 20 minutes or when prior clinical indications for the use of an anticoagulant exist (8). Traditionally, heparin is the anticoagulant used. However, as each patient responds differently to a dose of heparin, it is impossible to determine the timing of the peak effect of heparin, or when the plasma levels of heparin are diminished and the drug has 'worn off'. This problem is overcome by measuring the patient's blood's ability to clot – a test referred to as anticoagulant time (ACT) (6). Ideally, the arterial and venous sheaths should not be removed until the ACT level falls below 160 seconds (2; 11). Unfortunately, the ACT test loses its reliability below 225 seconds and many centres do not have easy access to an ACT monitor (6). Consequently, in many centres, heparin is allowed to dissipate naturally over 3–4 hours before the femoral sheaths are removed (11; 12).

Direct thrombin inhibitors such as bivalirudin are a new class of anticoagulant (10). Unlike heparin, the half-life of bivalirudin (25 minutes) is predictable in patients with a normal renal function. Although the half-life is longer in patients with renal failure, it takes approximately two half-lives for the drug levels to fall to a non-therapeutic level. Thus, sheaths can be safely removed in most patients 2 hours after bivalirudin has been discontinued (6). However, for patients on dialysis, it may take up to 8 hours before bivalirudin has reached a non-therapeutic level (2).

IS A HAEMATOMA PRESENT?

Poor insertion technique, vessel laceration or excessive anticoagulation may lead to problems such as haematoma formation prior to sheath removal. Large haematomas can cause considerable discomfort to the patient and have the potential to develop into false aneurysms (2). Haematomas in the soft tissue surrounding the site of the femoral sheath will feel firm and will have defined boundaries. If you are unsure whether one is present, compare it with the other thigh (8). If the haematoma is growing larger or there is a lot of oozing around the sheath, it should be removed earlier than planned (15).

WHAT IS THE PATIENT'S BLOOD PRESSURE?

If a patient is hypertensive (i.e. has a systolic blood pressure greater than 150 mmHg), the pressure within the arteries is high. This means that greater pressure is exerted at the arterial puncture site, impeding the clot's ability to adhere and seal off the puncture wound (13; 15). In addition to this, it increases the patient's risk of developing a haematoma (1). The patient's medication should be reviewed and if they are on anti-hypertensive drugs, these should be administered if the time is appropriate, to help reduce the patient's blood pressure before removing the femoral sheath (13). The doctor should be consulted, as the administration of glycerine trinitrate (GTN) either intravenously or orally will help to reduce the patient's blood pressure. As prolonged compression (greater than 30 minutes) will probably be required, the application of a compression device such as a FemoStop should be considered (2).

If a patient is hypotensive (i.e. with a systolic pressure of less than 100 mmHg), the patient is at risk of acute cerebral or myocardial ischaemia (12). The drugs used during the procedure can dilate the arteries, leading to a drop in blood pressure (2). In addition, the patient may be hypovolaemic, as they may have fasted prior to the procedure and the contrast agent encourages diuresis (8). The skin in such hypotensive patients usually feels normal or warm. They normally respond to the elevation of the lower extremities (more than 30°), as this increases venous return, and the administration of intravenous fluids (2; 8).

If the hypotension is drug-induced, the offending medication should be reversed or discontinued. This may mean stopping or decreasing the intravenous vasodilators, such as nitroglycerine, or administering naloxone if narcotics are found to be the cause of the drop in blood pressure (8).

WHAT IS THE PATIENT'S HEART RATE?

Iodinated contrast medium and/or a vasovagal response contribute to slowing of the heart rate (8). Therefore, in order to avoid a life-threatening bradyarrhythmia, it may be necessary to pre-medicate a symptomatic patient (one whose pulse is less than 50 beats per minute and whose systolic blood pressure is less than 100 mmHg) with 600 micrograms of atropine prior to removing the femoral sheaths (15). If a patient is asymptomatic but they have a heart rate of less than 50 beats per minute, their drug regime should be assessed, as drugs such as betablockers, calcium channel blockers, digoxin, amiodarone, methyldopa and clonidine may cause bradycardia (9).

POTENTIAL VASOVAGAL REACTIONS

Pressure on a large artery and pain can stimulate the vagus nerve, which will respond by slowing the heart rate and lowering blood pressure (8). Anxiety and tissue injury can also result in a vasovagal reaction (7). Early signs include pallor, nausea and/or yawning, vomiting, feeling hot or cold and shivering (7; 8). Vasovagal reactions may lead to irreversible shock if untreated. However, they respond dramatically to intravenous atropine (usual dose 0.6–1.0 mg). Elevation of the legs, infusion of gelatin (Gelofusine) and administering oxygen are helpful adjuncts (2; 8).

As vasovagal reactions may occur while pressing on the groin during sheath removal, it is advisable to have another person present who can administer treatment while pressure on the site is maintained (13).

CAN THE PATIENT LIE STILL?

If a patient has difficulty remaining immobile, the time to haemostasis may need to be lengthened (3; 13). Activity may dislodge the forming clot from the arterial puncture site and cause bleeding (3; 13).

IS THE PATIENT COMFORTABLE?

If the femoral sheaths are being removed several hours after the procedure, the local anaesthetic administered during the procedure will have worn off and removing the sheaths may be painful (15). Therefore, further lignocaine should be administered where the pressure is going to be applied. Hint: the lignocaine should be given early and while the anaesthetic is taking effect, other preparations can be completed (8). Systemic analgesia should be administered early if a patient develops a headache or backache due to prolonged bed rest. A bedpan or urinal should be offered to the patient before sheath removal, to promote the patient's comfort and reduce their movement immediately after sheath removal (13).

DOES THE PATIENT HAVE A VENOUS SHEATH IN SITU?

Occasionally, during cardiac intervention, an additional sheath will be inserted into the femoral vein to allow for a temporary pacing wire or venous access if peripheral venous access is a problem (8). When this does occur, the sheaths should be removed and haemostasis achieved separately in order to reduce the risk of atrioventricular fistula, haematoma formation and blood loss (8). If manual pressure is being used, the arterial sheath is usually removed first, then the venous sheath (2; 8).

ACHIEVING HAEMOSTASIS USING MANUAL PRESSURE

Manual pressure is also referred to as digital compression, as the operator presses on the puncture site with their fingers until haemostasis has been achieved (16).

The femoral sheath normally is inserted at a slight angle so that the arterial puncture site is not directly beneath the skin. Therefore, the operator should place their fingers over the femoral pulse, and not directly over the puncture site itself. Then, gentle pressure should be applied whilst removing the sheath. Care should be taken not to crush the sheath or to 'strip' clots into the distal artery. A small spurt of blood purges the arterial site of retained thrombi (8).

Firm downward pressure should then be applied. Five to ten minutes of pressure is usually suitable following cardiac catheterisation procedures such as coronary angiogram (12). However, the use of larger arterial sheaths, anticoagulants, glycoprotein (GP) IIb/IIIa inhibitors and antiplatelet agents in cardiac intervention procedures increases the risk of bleeding complications (2). Therefore, 15–20 minutes of firm pressure should be applied following these procedures. After the first 10 minutes of firm compression, the pressure should be gradually released until the haemostasis is achieved. During the pressure application, the pedal pulses should be checked every 2–3 minutes, to ensure that the distal pulses are not obliterated completely (8; 12). In addition to this, the operator should be feeling for haematoma formation, as this indicates that it is bleeding under the skin and they may need to readjust the position of where they are applying the pressure.

The venous sheath is removed in a similar fashion but 5–10 minutes of pressure is usually sufficient (8).

Once haemostasis has been achieved, the patient must remain on bed rest. The typical recommendation is to lie flat for 1 hour and sit up for 1 hour when a size 5 French catheter has been used. The patient should lie flat for 2 hours and sit up for 1–2 hours if a size 6 French sheath or larger catheter has been used (4; 16).

MECHANICAL COMPRESSION

The disadvantages of manual compression are that it is time-consuming and uncomfortable for the operator, since a reasonable degree of force is required. As a result, a number of mechanical devices have been tried. These include sandbags, mechanical C-Clamps, stasis buttons and pneumatic devices. It has been found that sandbags do not reduce vascular complications and may even increase patient discomfort. The mechanical clamps and pneumatic devices have been shown to be as effective as manual pressure in preventing complications; however, compression time may be longer (12).

To prevent complications, these devices should be applied by trained individuals following the manufacturer's instructions. The patient should be monitored frequently, as misalignment of the device and puncture site may result in bleeding or haematoma. Excessive pressure on the femoral artery may deprive the leg of oxygenated blood, resulting in limb ischaemia (8).

FEMOSTOP PRESSURE SYSTEM

The FemoStop is an example of a pneumatic compression device. It consists of an air-filled, clear plastic compression bubble that moulds to the skin contours. It is held in place by a strap passed around the hips. The clear plastic dome allows the operator to see the puncture site. The amount of pressure applied by the FemoStop depends on the patient's own blood pressure and is controlled using a sphygmo-manometer gauge. A FemoStop can be applied prior to removing the femoral sheaths, or when bleeding persists despite prolonged manual pressure (8; 14).

A STEP-BY-STEP GUIDE TO REMOVING A FEMORAL SHEATH USING A FEMOSTOP

1. Examine the puncture site carefully.
2. Note and mark the edges of any haematoma.
3. Record the patient's current blood pressure.
4. Identify the arterial puncture site by feeling for the femoral pulse. Some operators like to mark it in ink.
5. Place the belt under the patient's hips. The belt should be in line with the puncture site and equally aligned either side of the patient.
6. Attach the dome to the FemoStop arch and peel back the lid. Keep the dome sterile.
7. Connect the dome to the pressure pump and close the valve.
8. Align the centre of the star on the FemoStop pressure dome over the arterial puncture site. Attach the belt to the arch and tighten slowly to ensure the arch remains level and square and the dome remains perpendicular to the arterial puncture.
9. The belt should fit snugly, but not be too tight.
10. If present, the venous sheath is usually removed first when a FemoStop system is used for compression.
11. To remove a venous sheath, inflate the dome to 20–30 mmHg and remove the sheath.
12. If bleeding persists, slowly increase the pressure until haemostasis is achieved. Achieving haemostasis in the venous puncture site before removing the arterial sheath minimises the formation of arteriovenous fistula.
13. For the arterial sheath, inflate the dome to 60–80 mmHg and remove the sheath. Increase the pressure in the dome to 10–20 mmHg above the systolic blood pressure.
14. Maintain full compression for 3 minutes.
15. Reduce pressure in the dome to medium blood pressure. After appropriate duration, per hospital protocol, lower the pressure by 10–20 mmHg every

few minutes until the pressure is zero. During this time, it is important
to monitor the pedal pulse to ensure that the leg is not being deprived of
oxygenated blood.
16. The FemoStop can be left in place at low pressure, if appropriate.
17. If there is no sign of bleeding or haematoma formation, release the air from
    the FemoStop dome.
18. Roll the FemoStop dome off the puncture site.
19. The patient can sit up 10–15 minutes after this if there is no sign of bleeding
    or haematoma (8; 14).

The preparations for removing a femoral sheath using a FemoStop are the same
as those for using manual compression. Therefore, the following care plan could
be followed up to step 14.

CARE PLANS

The aim is to remove the femoral sheath(s) using manual compression, obtain
haemostasis at the puncture site and prevent complications.

	Nursing action	Rationale and key points
1	Using an aseptic technique, prepare a trolley with the required equipment (see Box 1)	Reduces risk of cross-infection. Easily available equipment saves time (5)
2	Explain and discuss the procedure with the patient	Ensures that the patient understands the procedure and gives his or her consent (5)
3	Place the patient in a supine position and with the head of the bed elevated less than 10°	Allows better access to the site and the location of landmarks (8)
4	Check the colour, movement, sensation and pulses in both legs. Mark the location of the pulses	To obtain a baseline for comparison after the sheath is removed (11)
5	Ensure that the patient has intravenous access	Allows emergency intravenous medication to be administered (8)
6	Check that cardiac monitoring is properly attached	To observe heart rhythm and rate during sheath removal (11)
7	Set the non-invasive automatic blood-pressure cuff to check blood pressure every 3 minutes	Pressure on a large artery and pain may stimulate the vagus nerve to slow heart rate and lower blood pressure (8; 13)

	Nursing action	Rationale and key points
8	Clean hands with a bactericidal skin-cleanser solution	Contamination may result from handling outer packets (5)
9	Apply protective equipment, as in hospital protocol, such as apron, gloves, goggles, mask	To reduce the risk of being contaminated by the accidental spurting of the patient's blood and cross-infection (5; 8)
10	Remove semi-occlusive dressing and tape from sheath site. If a haematoma is noted, mark the border outline	To enable easy removal of the sheath(s) and assess any increase in size of the haematoma (5; 13)
11	Clean sheath site with sterile gauze	Achieves clean field of vision of suture and sheath site (13)
12	Locate femoral pulse proximal to insertion site. Position three fingers of left hand sequentially up artery, starting from puncture site, until arterial pulse can be palpated	The femoral sheath is inserted at an angle; therefore, the actual puncture in the artery is 1–2 cm above the puncture site towards the head (8)
13	Infiltrate 5 ml prescribed 1 or 2% lignocaine on either side of the femoral artery, maximum dose 10 ml, to the area in which pressure will be applied	Lignocaine is a topical anaesthetic that renders the area in which it was administered insensitive to pain by blocking the nerve impulses that transmit pain (9)
14	Cut the retaining suture	The suture is used to secure the sheath to the patient (2)
15	If there is both an arterial and venous sheath, you should prepare to remove the arterial sheath first	Reduces peripheral vascular complications (8)
16	As previously, locate femoral pulse; place fingers on pressure position; while pressing firmly, gently remove the sheath from the artery; do not crush the sheath	Crushing the sheath may 'strip' a clot into the distal artery (8)
17	Relax pressure enough to allow a small spurt of blood	This action purges any retained thrombi (8)
18	Manual pressure is held firmly for 15–20 minutes: 5 minutes' full pressure; 5 minutes' 75% pressure; 5 minutes' 50% pressure; 5 minutes' 25% pressure	Pressure controls bleeding and promotes haemostasis. Up to a further 10 minutes of pressure may be required when the patient is on antiplatelet therapy (8)

Nursing action	Rationale and key points
19 During compression, check pedal pulse every 3–5 minutes	The pedal pulse may decrease during application of full pressure, but should not disappear. If pulse is absent, pressure over the femoral artery should be lowered to allow distal circulation (8)
20 While applying reduced pressure with one hand, palpate the surrounding area with the other to detect haematoma formation. Skin should be soft and pliable	A haematoma will feel firm and have a defined boundary (8)
21 If a haematoma begins to form, check to be sure your hand is positioned properly	Appropriate compression can disperse and reduce a haematoma (2)
22 After holding for 20 minutes, slowly release pressure and observe for bleeding or haematoma formation	Ensures that haemostasis has been achieved (13)

- 5–10 ml lignocaine
- Stitch cutter
- Gauze
- Sterile gloves
- Ink marker
- 10 ml saline flush
- 600 micrograms atropine
- 1 litre Gelofusine and blood-giving set
- Oxygen mask attached to oxygen administration set
- FemoStop equipment (13)

Box 1. Equipment needed for femoral sheath removal

NURSING CARE FOLLOWING FEMORAL SHEATH REMOVAL

While the patient is on bed rest, the nurse should maintain half-hourly observations on the patient, checking the following:

- the pulse and blood pressure for signs of hypovolaemic shock;
- the affected groin to ensure no recurrence of bleeding or haematoma formation;
- pedal pulses, skin colour and warmth on the affected leg's foot to ensure that no distal ischaemia has occurred (3).

In addition to this, patients are advised to:

- Keep the affected leg straight for the first 2 hours if manual pressure was used.
- Press on the groin site when coughing or sneezing.
- Call for nurse's assistance if there is a recurrence of bleeding.
- Inform the nurse if they experience chest pain.
- Drink plenty of fluids in order to prevent hypotension (11).

REFERENCES

1. Anderson, K., Bregendahl, M., Kaestel, H., Skriver, M. and Ravkilde, J. (2005) 'Haematoma after coronary angiography and percutaneous coronary intervention via the femoral artery frequency and risk factors', *European Journal of Cardiovascular Nursing*, **4**(2): 123–7.
2. Baim, D. S. (2006) *Grossman's Cardiac Catheterisation: Angiography and Intervention*, 7th edn, Philadelphia, PA, Lippincott Williams & Wilkins.
3. Botti, M., Williamson, B. and Steen, K. (2001) 'Coronary angiography observations: Evidence-based or ritualistic practice?', *Heart Lung*, **30**(2): 138–45.
4. Braunweld, E., Zipes, D. and Libby, P. (2001) *Heart Disease: A Textbook of Cardiovascular Medicine*, Vol. 1, 6th edn, London, W.B. Saunders Co.
5. Dougherty, L. and Lister, S. (2004) *The Royal Marsden Hospital of Clinical Nursing Procedures*, 6th edn, Oxford, Blackwell Publishing.
6. Galli, G. (2005) 'Ask the experts: Re removing arterial and venous sheaths after PCI', *Critical Care Nurse*, available online at *www.findarticles.com*.
7. Hadaway, L. (2001) 'I.V. Rounds: Managing a vasovagal reaction', *Nursing*, April, available online at *www.springnet.com*.
8. Kern, M. (2003) *The Cardiac Catheterisation Handbook*, 4th edn, London, Mosby.
9. Lilley, L. and Aucker, R. (2001) *Pharmacology and the Nursing Process*, 3rd edn, London, Mosby.
10. Montalsecot, G., Andersen, H., Antoniucer, D., Betriu, A., de Boer, M., Grip, L., *et al.* (2004) 'Recommendations on percutaneous coronary intervention for the reperfusion of acute ST elevation myocardial infarction', *Heart*, 90, available online at *http://heart.bmjjournals.com/cgi/content/full/90/6/e37*.
11. Morton, P. G., Fontaine, D. K., Hudak, C. M. and Gallo, B. M. (2005) *Critical Care Nursing: A Holistic Approach*, 8th edn, Philadelphia, PA, Lippincott Williams & Wilkins.
12. Norell, M. and Perrins, J. (2003) *Essential Interventional Cardiology*, Philadelphia, PA, W.B. Saunders Co.
13. O'Grady, E. (2002) 'Removal of a femoral sheath following PTCA in cardiac patients', *Professional Nurse*, **17**(11): 651–4.
14. Radi Medical Inc. (2003) 'FemoStop II: Femoral compression system, pocket guide', available online at *www.radi.se*.
15. Swanton, R. H. (2003) *Pocket Consultant Cardiology*, 5th edn, Oxford, Blackwell Publishing.
16. Tagney, J. and Lackie, D. (2005) 'Bed-rest post femoral arterial sheath removal: What is safe practice? A clinical audit', British Association of Critical Care Nurses, *Nursing in Critical Care*, **10**(4): 167–73.
17. Topol, E. (1999) *Textbook of Interventional Cardiology*, 3rd edn, Philadelphia, PA, W. B. Saunders Co.

3 Complications Associated with Percutaneous Coronary Procedures

Although complications associated with cardiac catheterisation and intervention procedures are relatively few, these procedures are not entirely risk-free. It has been found that older people, women, diabetics and those with impaired renal function, unstable angina, congestive heart failure, left main coronary artery-equivalent disease and multi-vessel multi-lesion coronary artery disease have an increased risk of complications (5). The complication rates associated with each procedure will be discussed in their respective chapters; this chapter will look at the individual complications in a little more detail.

The majority of studies looking at complications associated with cardiac catheterisation or intervention involved coronary angiograms and percutaneous coronary interventions (PCIs). However, the studies showed that the most commonly encountered complications related to vascular access and radiographic contrast media (15). Therefore, the nurse should be familiar with potential complications, no matter which coronary procedure or intervention the patient is undergoing.

DEATH

The mortality rates associated with coronary catheterisation and intervention procedures are low (11). Procedure-related mortality associated with diagnostic catheterisation is 0.1% (i.e. one in 1,000) (2). The BCIS (2004) audit showed that in the United Kingdom, the mortality rate for PCI was 0.56%. This was sub-divided and acutely ill patients with acute coronary syndrome and non-ST-elevated myocardial infarction patients accounted for three-quarters of this mortality (3).

CORONARY ARTERY BYPASS GRAFT (CABG)

Major complications associated with PCI were arterial thrombus forming on the site of the vessel injury, which might occur alone or in association with coronary artery dissection. If these complications occurred, the patient previously required emergency coronary artery bypass graft (CABG) surgery (14). However, the use of coronary artery stents and glycoprotein (GP) IIb/IIIa inhibitors has considerably reduced these problems and, now, fewer than 1% of PCI patients undergo emergency CABG surgery (14).

PERFORATION OF THE CORONARY ARTERY

Perforation of the coronary artery is very rare during PCI but may be caused by the guidewire or the use of an excessively large stent. Although emergency CABG surgery may be necessary, it can be dealt with by implanting a covered stent to seal off the perforation (16).

GUIDEWIRE FRACTURE

Although it is a very rare complication, if the guidewire used in the procedure were to break off in the patient's body, it would have to be retrieved surgically (16).

ANGINA

Angina is a discomfort in the chest and adjacent areas due to the transiently inadequate blood supply to the heart (8). Therefore, some degree of angina is anticipated during PCI procedures, as the affected coronary artery will be temporarily occluded when the angioplasty balloon is being inflated. This chest pain is usually relieved by intra-coronary nitroglycerine or the removal of the balloon dilation catheter (11). It may also occur after the procedure due to paroxysmal tachycardia in the ischaemic patient. It usually responds to sublingual nitroglycerine and sedation. The electrocardiogram should be checked and if the angina recurs, the patient should be monitored. Occasionally, intravenous analgesia such as diamorphine is required (16).

MYOCARDIAL INFARCTION AND CORONARY ARTERY SPASM

Persistent chest pain after the procedure, reflected in changes in heart rate, blood pressure and elevated ST segments, indicates that the patient has probably occluded a major coronary artery due to a thrombus or dissection. Very occasionally, it may be due to coronary spasm. Intravenous analgesia should be administered and intravenous nitrates commenced (16). Coronary artery spasm sometimes requires emergency surgical intervention (CABG) when the vasoconstriction, occlusion or ischaemia cannot be reversed through the administration of nitrates (11).

ACUTE CLOSURE OF THE CORONARY ARTERY

Acute closure of the coronary artery may be defined as the occlusion of the coronary artery occurring during or after the coronary artery dilation, with consequent electrocardiographic and haemodynamic instability. It is the most common cause of peri-procedural myocardial infarction, referral for CABG surgery and death (12). Acute closure occurs in approximately 3% of those undergoing angioplasty. An estimated 70–80% of acute closures occur while the patient is still in the catheterisation laboratory (cath lab), but a significant proportion occur afterwards, within 6 hours of the procedure. Acute closure of the coronary artery is rare 6 hours after PCI and very unlikely after 24 hours (11; 12).

Acute closure can be caused by coronary artery dissection, coronary artery spasm and thrombus formation. Treatment options include immediate repeat balloon dilation, emergency CABG surgery or pharmacological therapy (11).

CORONARY ARTERY DISSECTION

A dissection occurs when the inner lining of the coronary artery separates from the middle layer, which may peel back, thus blocking the coronary artery. This could cause a major obstruction, leading to a deterioration in blood flow which would result in severe ischaemia or myocardial infarction and would require emergency CABG surgery if the cardiologist was unable to stent it (11). It is believed that the vigorous injection of the contrast dye against an atherosclerotic plaque may cause a coronary artery dissection, in rare cases, during an angiogram. In addition to this, it may be caused by trauma from the tip of the catheter in the ostium of the coronary artery (2). However, coronary artery dissection occurs more often during a PCI, as the inflation of the balloon may cause the inner layer of the coronary wall to split (11).

BALLOON RUPTURE

Rupture of the catheter balloon may occur with or without stents, and may be the result of rough handling of the balloon before introducing it into the guide catheter or during manual mounting of the stent. The most common type of balloon rupture is a pinhole perforation, but this type of rupture can cause a dissection. During inflation, the very high pressure in the balloon forces a tiny powerful jet of contrast into the wall of the artery, resulting in a dissection. Sudden explosive bursting of a balloon may result in vessel perforation. Other consequences of balloon rupture include air embolism and trapping of the burst balloon when it becomes enmeshed in a partially deployed stent. If it does occur, it is important to monitor and treat any complications (12).

CEREBRAL VASCULAR INFARCTION

Although cerebral vascular infarction rarely occurs during cardiac catheterisation procedures or interventions, it is considered a major complication (9). The use of anticoagulants during the procedure increases the chances of an at-risk patient's suffering a cerebral bleed (12). Alternatively, if a thrombus occurs during the procedure, it may travel to the brain, resulting in a cerebral vascular infarction (9).

ARRHYTHMIAS

Serious arrhythmias (including ventricular fibrillation, ventricular tachycardia, supraventricular tachycardia, asystole and heart block) occur in approximately 1% of either right-sided or left-sided heart catheterisations. In almost all instances, the arrhythmia can be managed successfully by prompt recognition and treatment (9). In general, serious ventricular arrhythmias occur in two situations: 1. Excessive catheter manipulation within the left or right ventricular chambers, especially when the myocardium is more prone to irritability; the arrhythmia may resolve by removing the catheter. 2. The reduction of oxygenated blood to the right coronary artery when the ionic contrast dye is being injected may induce ventricular fibrillation; this incidence can be reduced by injecting the smallest amount of contrast agent needed to opacify the arterial tree (2). If a life-threatening arrhythmia such as a ventricular tachycardia or ventricular fibrillation occurs, it requires immediate defibrillation (9; 11).

The following may increase the patient's risk of a tachyarrhythmia:

1. Some sedative agents used during the procedure may cause arrhythmias (9).
2. Low levels of potassium (hypokalaemia) in the patient's blood increase the excitability and sensitivity of the myocardium (11).
3. The cardiac muscle becomes irritable when the flow of oxygen-rich blood decreases, as happens for a controlled period of time during the placement and inflation of the dilation balloon across the lesion during a PCI (11).

Ischaemia induced by injecting the right coronary artery with ionic contrast dye may cause bradycardia (a ventricular heart rate of less than 60 beats per minute). Patients should be treated with intravenous atropine sulphate, 0.6–1 mg every 5 minutes to a maximum dose of 3 mg. A temporary pacemaker is rarely needed to treat this bradycardia (9). However, patients with bundle branch block are prone to bradyarrhythmias during cardiac catheterisation or intervention and therefore may need to have a temporary pacemaker during the procedure (9).

HYPOTENSION

Hypotension can be defined as a blood pressure of less than 90 mmHg or a 25–30% decrease in systolic blood pressure from the resting baseline values (11).

Hypotension following PCI is not uncommon but should be vigorously investigated and treated, because hypotension from any cause may decrease coronary blood flow. This may cause cerebral or myocardial ischaemia, or induce a blood clot to be formed in the recently dilated artery (12; 17). As almost all available stents are made of thrombotic material, the low blood pressure may enable the blood to stick to the stent and form a thrombus (12).

Patients may develop hypotension after cardiac catheterisation or intervention as a result of dehydration because they fasted before the procedure and radiographic contrast dye acts as an osmotic diuretic (17). Therefore, patients should be encouraged to drink plenty of fluids after the procedure, as such hypotension usually resolves after the radiographic contrast dye is 'washed out' of the circulation by way of the kidneys (2). If the patient is unable to drink, then they should receive intravenous fluids and the foot end of the bed should be elevated (more than 30°), as this increases venous return (2; 9).

If the hypotension is drug-induced, the offending medication should be reversed or discontinued. This may mean stopping or decreasing the intravenous vasodilators, such as nitroglycerine, or administering naloxone if narcotics are found to be the cause of the drop in blood pressure (9). Other causes of symptomatic hypotension include myocardial ischaemia, cardiac tamponade, gastrointestinal or retroperitoneal bleeding, arterial puncture bleeding and a vasovagal reaction to a haematoma after the procedure (2; 9).

As blood pressure may drop when a person stands up abruptly after a prolonged bed rest, the patient should be advised to take things slowly when they begin to mobilise following the procedure (17).

VASOVAGAL REACTIONS

Pressure on a large artery and pain can stimulate the vagus nerve, which will respond by slowing the heart rate and lowering blood pressure (9). Anxiety and tissue injury can also result in a vasovagal reaction (7). Early signs include pallor, nausea and/or yawning, vomiting, feeling hot or cold and shivering (7; 9). Vasovagal reactions may lead to irreversible shock if untreated. However, they respond dramatically to intravenous atropine (usual dose 0.6–1.0 mg). Elevation of the legs, infusion of a colloid (e.g. Gelofusine) and administering oxygen are helpful adjuncts (2; 9).

As vasovagal reactions may occur while pressing on the groin during sheath removal, it is advisable to have another person present who can administer treatment while pressure on the site is maintained (13).

BLEEDING/HAEMORRHAGE

Bleeding may occur at the arterial puncture site or at a distant accidental puncture site. In addition to this, bleeding may occur spontaneously at a remote site, such as a gastric bleed or cerebral bleed as a result of the heavy anticoagulation. Bleeding complications tend to be noticed after the procedure (12).

Procedures that require larger catheters such as directional coronary atherectomy, rotational atherectomy and the use of intra-aortic balloon pumping increase the risk of patients' developing bleeding complications at the arterial puncture site. The use of post-procedural heparin and IIb/IIIa antagonists also increases the patient's risk of bleeding. As the majority of the bleeding usually occurs at the arterial puncture site, it can normally be controlled by manual compression. Clamping devices such as FemoStops may be used, but need to be applied carefully by experienced staff to be effective (12).

STOPPING BLEEDING FROM AN ARTERIAL PUNCTURE

Bleeding from the femoral, brachial or radial artery is controlled by applying firm pressure. If the bleeding is not controlled after 30 minutes:

• Check the clotting screen. If the patient is on warfarin, fresh frozen plasma may help. Vitamin K is not usually recommended, as it makes subsequent anticoagulation very difficult. If the patient has just had heparin, then check the activated partial thromboplastin time (APTT), as protamine reversal may help (dose of protamine: 10 mg/1,000 units of heparin administered).
• Check the patient's blood pressure, as a high systolic pressure will exacerbate bleeding. Administering nitrates will help to reduce the hypertension (16).

HAEMATOMAS

A haematoma occurs when the arterial puncture site is not sealed properly and blood accumulates in the surrounding tissue (12). This is the most frequent complication that occurs when the femoral artery puncture site is used for coronary angiography and PCI (1). In order to monitor the growth of a haematoma, the outer edges should be marked with washable marker pen, then firm pressure should be applied just above the skin puncture on the artery. As haematomas are very tender, analgesia should be administered (4). Clamping devices such as FemoStops may be used, but need to be applied carefully by experienced staff to be effective. It is important to catch haemorrhage early before a large haematoma has developed, as compression becomes difficult and ineffective once there is a large, boggy mass. This especially applies to clamping devices (12).

If the patient loses a lot of blood into the surrounding tissue, they may require a blood transfusion. In addition to this, the haematoma may need to be removed surgically (4; 11). Fortunately, the majority of haematomas after cardiac catheterisation procedures do not need such intervention (1). The blood in the surrounding tissue as a result of a haematoma will break down and be reabsorbed by the body (12). But this process takes several weeks and the resulting bruising may appear to expand and change colour from dark blue to greenish yellow. The haematoma may compress the femoral nerve, which, in turn, may make the leg muscle feel weak, with an unpleasant tingling sensation in the leg. This may make it difficult for the patient to walk normally for several months (1).

As the brachial artery cutdown is usually repaired by direct suture at the end of the procedure, bleeding is often venous oozing only, which will respond to direct pressure. Haematoma development in the arm can be observed by measuring the arm's circumference and may require exploring and re-suturing of the brachial artery (16).

Several factors were identified that increased a patient's risk of developing a haematoma. These include:

- treatments with low-molecular-weight heparin (LMWH) and GPIIb/IIIa inhibitors;
- steroid treatment;
- a systolic blood pressure of more than 160 mmHg in conjunction with a coronary angiogram was associated with a 3.6 times (or higher) risk of developing a haematoma;
- changing personnel during manual compression;
- the most significant risk factor is the arterial puncture itself (1).

PSEUDOANEURYSM

A pseudoaneurysm is also known as a false aneurysm. It occurs when there is inadequate compression of the arterial puncture site following a percutaneous cardiac procedure. The resultant haematoma is encapsulated and maintains a connection to the artery (2). Therefore, the presence of a hard, tender pulsatile lump with bruit over the puncture site is a good indicator that a false aneurysm has developed. The diagnosis can be confirmed by ultrasound imaging (16).

Pseudoaneurysms may resolve spontaneously, particularly in patients who are not anticoagulated, but they may increase in size, especially in anticoagulated patients. Increased painful swelling may compress the femoral nerve and may rupture, increasing blood loss; therefore, in the past, all femoral pseudoaneurysms were routinely repaired by the vascular surgeon (9; 12). Nowadays, with ultrasound imaging techniques, these false channels can be easily identified and non-surgical closure selected. Using ultrasound guidance, thrombin or collagen can be injected directly into the aneurysm forming a blood clot, thus sealing it (2; 9). Alternatively, firm pressure with an ultrasound probe on the neck of the aneurysm for about 20–30 minutes can result in the false aneurysm's thrombosing. A compression device such as a FemoStop can be used on the ward as an alternative. The majority of femoral false aneurysms can be dealt with in this way if the neck of the false aneurysm is small. It is painful and the patient will need sedation and analgesia (16).

RETROPERITONEAL HAEMATOMA

A retroperitoneal haematoma is when a patient bleeds behind the peritoneum (i.e. into the abdominal and pelvic cavities) (9). Although it is a rare complication, it is potentially fatal, as bleeding into the retroperitoneal area can go undetected for quite some time because the cavity is so large (4). Retroperitoneal bleeding should be suspected in patients with hypotension, tachycardia, pallor, a rapid fall in their full blood count after the procedure, lower abdominal or back pain, or neurologic changes in the leg in which the puncture was made. High femoral artery puncture and full anticoagulation increase the patient's risk of a retroperitoneal bleed (9).

The diagnosis can be confirmed with abdominal ultrasound or computed tomography (CT) examination. Anticoagulation should be stopped and reversed if necessary with protamine and fresh frozen plasma, despite the risk of acute coronary closure in certain patients. Hypovolaemia should be promptly corrected. Surgical intervention is rarely indicated (12).

ARTERIOVENOUS FISTULA

An arteriovenous fistula is an abnormal direct connection between the artery and the vein and can occur if both the artery and the vein are cannulated on the same side for the procedure. This is particularly the case if the vein runs superficially to the artery. Most heal spontaneously but they are also amenable to compression treatment similar to that for a pseudoaneurysm. Arteriovenous fistulae may be avoided if the puncture sites are made 1 cm or more apart (12). In addition to this, the arterial and venous sheaths should be removed separately and haemostasis acquired prior to removing the other sheath (13).

RENAL NEPHROPATHY

The radio-opaque contrast material used during cardiac catheterisation and intervention procedures is a hyperosmotic solution that is filtered and excreted by the kidneys. High doses of the radio-opaque contrast can cause acute renal failure, in which the patient requires dialysis (11). This is known as contrast-induced nephropathy.

Contrast-induced nephropathy has been defined as 'an impairment of renal function manifesting 1–3 days subsequent to contrast administration in the absence of an alternative aetiology' (6). Risk factors predicting the likelihood of contrast-induced nephropathy include pulmonary oedema, arterial repair, a neurological event, diabetes, peripheral or cerebral vascular diseases, the volume of contrast used and renal impairment or failure (6).

Checking blood for urea and electrolytes prior to the procedure is important, as raised levels of serum creatinine are an indicator of problems with kidney function. With such patients, good hydration is important, so at-risk patients may have intravenous saline before and/or after the procedure. In addition, depending on the cardiologist's preference, they may receive adjunctive therapies such as adenosine receptor antagonist, endothelin antagonists and N-acetylcysteine. The most promising and widely used of these is N-acetylcysteine (6).

Metformin is not nephrotoxic but is contraindicated in patients with renal failure because it may result in serious lactic acidosis. In patients without renal failure, it can be used up to the day of contrast administration but should be withheld thereafter for 48 hours or until serum creatinine returns to normal (6). In addition to this, nephrotoxic drugs and non-steroidal anti-inflammatory drugs should be avoided for a few days prior to the procedure (6).

INFECTIONS/FEBRILE EPISODES

As with any intravenous procedure, percutaneous catheterisation or intervention can cause phlebitis, bacteraemia and infection. As the procedure is carried out under sterile conditions, this is very rare. However, the infection rate is greater with repeated use of the same groin site. Therefore, patients who undergo two or three procedures within a few weeks are at a greater risk of infection (4). Leaving the femoral sheath in situ for a prolonged period of time (1–5 days) also increases the patient's risk of infection (9). In addition to this, haematomas may provide a site for infection (12).

Post-catheterisation pyrexia is usually due to a dye reaction and settles within 24 hours. Persisting pyrexia, however, should be investigated and treated along the usual lines with blood cultures, urine cultures, etc. prior to antibiotics (16).

CONTRAST SENSITIVITY/DYE REACTION

Patients with known contrast allergy should be given either oral or intravenous prophylaxis 24 hours before the procedure (15). The signs and symptoms of contrast sensitivity are usually mild; however, they include anxiety, skin reactions, blushing, itchiness, urticaria, blisters, nausea and vomiting, laryngospasm, headache, hypotension, pyrexia and rigors. Very rarely, it causes more severe reactions: fits, anaphylactic shock and transient cortical disturbance, such as cortical blindness (11; 16):

- Urticaria and skin reactions are usually helped by intravenous antihistamines and, in more severe cases, by additional intravenous hydrocortisone.
- Nausea and vomiting can be treated with intravenous antiemetics.
- Hypotension should be treated with intravenous fluids, especially in patients who have been excessively diuresed or who have had a lot of dye.
- Pyrexia and rigors are usually transient. Rest and sedation are all that are necessary.

- Anaphylactic shock usually occurs in the cath lab rather than on the ward, and should be treated by urgent volume replacement with intravenous plasma substitute or normal saline, hydrocortisone and adrenaline.
- Cortical disturbances are rare and, again, usually transient. They are not necessarily embolic, and may in part be due to vascular spasm or an osmotic effect of the dye.
- Fits are controlled as in grand mal epilepsy with intravenous diazepam (16).

EMBOLISMS

Developing an embolism after cardiac catheterisation or intervention is a relatively rare complication (11). If the emboli lodge distal to the puncture site, they can be readily recognised by loss of peripheral pulse and skin mottling (9), which is why the limb distal to the puncture site should be checked regularly after the procedure. They can be treated surgically (thrombectomy), unless the area affected is small, in which case it may be treated conservatively with heparin. Thrombotic emboli are more commonly associated with using an intra-aortic balloon pump, in which case, the balloon should be removed (12).

On a rare occasion, the cholesterol in the coronary arteries might be dislodged during the procedure, which would cause problems if it lodged elsewhere in the body. Therefore, medical staff should be informed if the patient complains of headache, abdominal ache, not passing urine or lung haemorrhage (9).

LOST RADIAL PULSE FOLLOWING BRACHIAL ARTERY CATHETERISATION

The loss of radial pulse following brachial artery catheterisation is very rare and occurs in fewer than 1% of brachial artery punctures. Ideally, it should be treated in the cath lab at the time. A few patients will regain the radial pulse when they warm up and brachial spasm regresses. A numb hand may occur in the presence of a good radial pulse. This is usually the effect of the lignocaine on the median nerve at the catheter site and sensation returns within 12 hours. Residual median nerve damage is rare and probably due to unnecessary manipulation of the nerve during the catheterisation procedure (16).

LOST FEMORAL PULSE FOLLOWING FEMORAL ARTERY CATHETERISATION

A loss of the foot pulse following femoral artery catheterisation is also rare, but may be transient (24 hours) in children. In adults, however, loss of the foot pulse is usually irreversible and requires femoral thrombectomy (16).

PERICARDIAL TAMPONADE

The heart is surrounded by a triple-layered bag called the pericardium (or pericardial sac). It maintains the heart's position in the chest and allows sufficient movement for vigorous and rapid contraction. The outer layer is a fibrous, tough, inelastic tissue (18). The pericardial sac normally holds about 25 ml of pericardial fluid, which cushions and protects the heart and reduces friction between the membranes of the heart (11).

Bleeding into the pericardial sac or a small pericardial rupture may or may not cause cardiac tamponade, depending on the amount of pressure in the pericardium (11). However, an increase of 50–100 ml of blood or more into the pericardium may compress the heart and thus decrease cardiac filling, which leads to reduced cardiac output and, eventually, shock (11). This should be considered in any patient who becomes hypotensive, breathless and anuretic following catheterisation (11). It is a very rare complication of routine cardiac catheterisation or intervention, but it is a recognised complication of the trans-septal puncture procedure or right-ventricle biopsy. Diagnosis is confirmed by echocardiography. Pericardial aspiration may be required (16).

SIGNS AND SYMPTOMS OF CARDIAC TAMPONADE

The signs and symptoms of cardiac tamponade are:

- paradoxical pulse;
- narrowed pulse pressure, hypotension;
- tachycardia;
- weak peripheral pulse;
- distant, muffled heart sounds;
- jugular venous distension;
- high central venous pressure;
- decreased level of consciousness;
- low urine output;
- cool, mottled skin (10).

X-RAY DURING PREGNANCY

Elective cardiac catheterisation and intervention procedures are contraindicated during pregnancy, as the x-ray radiation increases the risk of fetal central nerve damage, growth retardation, malformation or miscarriage. As direct irradiation of the uterus can usually be avoided in procedures that involve structures above the diaphragm, cardiac catheterisation and interventions can be justified in an emergency. Extra precautions will be taken during fluoroscopy (2).

REFERENCES

1. Anderson, K., Bregendahl, M., Kaestel, H., Skriver, M. and Ravkilde, J. (2005) 'Haematoma after coronary angiography and percutaneous coronary intervention via the femoral artery frequency and risk factors', *European Journal of Cardiovascular Nursing*, **4**(2): 123–7.
2. Baim, D. S. (2006) *Grossman's Cardiac Catheterisation: Angiography and Intervention*, 7th edn, Philadelphia, PA, Lippincott Williams & Wilkins.
3. BCIS (2004) 'The British Cardiac Intervention Society audit for PCI', available online at *www.bcis.org.uk*.
4. Beattie, S. (1999) 'Cut the risks for cardiac cath patients', *RN*, **62**(1): 50–5.
5. Braunweld, E., Zipes, D. and Libby, P. (2001) *Heart Disease: A Textbook of Cardiovascular Medicine*, Vol. 1, 6th edn, London, W. B. Saunders Co.
6. Brinker, J. A., Davidson, C. J. and Laskey, W. (2005) 'Preventing in-hospital cardiac and renal complications in high-risk PCI patients', *European Heart Journal Supplement*, **7**(Suppl G): G13–25, available online at *www.eurheartj/sui054*.
7. Hadaway, L. (2001) 'I. V. rounds: Managing a vasovagal reaction', *Nursing*, April: 73, available online at *www.springnet.com*.
8. Julian, D. G., Cowan, J. C. and McLenachan, J. M. (2005) *Cardiology*, 8th edn, London, Elsevier Saunders.
9. Kern, M. (2003) *The Cardiac Catheterisation Handbook*, 4th edn, London, Mosby.
10. Lemone, P. and Burke, K. (2004) *Medical/Surgical Nursing: Critical Thinking in Client Care*, 3rd edn, Upper Saddle River, NJ, Prentice Hall.
11. Morton, P. G., Fontaine, D. K., Hudak, C. M. and Gallo, B. M. (2005) *Critical Care Nursing: A Holistic Approach*, 8th edn, Philadelphia, PA, Lippincott Williams & Wilkins.
12. Norell, M. and Perrins, J. (2003) *Essential Interventional Cardiology*, Philadelphia, PA, W.B. Saunders Co.
13. O'Grady, E. (2002) 'Removal of a femoral sheath following coronary angioplasty in cardiac patients', *Professional Nurse*, **19**(11): 651–4.
14. Popma, J. J., Berger, P., Ohman, E. M., Harrington, R. A., Grines, C. and Weitz, J. I. (2004) 'The Seventh ACCP Conference on Antithrombotic and Thrombolytic Therapy', *Chest*, **126**(3 Suppl): 575S–99S.
15. Rosendorff C. (2005) *Essential Cardiology: Principles and Practice*, 2nd edn, Totowa, NJ, Humana Press.
16. Swanton, R. H. (2003) *Pocket Consultant Cardiology*, 5th edn, Oxford, Blackwell Publishing.
17. Topol, E. (1999) *Textbook of Interventional Cardiology*, 3rd edn, Philadelphia, PA, W.B. Saunders Co.
18. Tortora, G. J. and Derrickson, B. (2006) *Principles of Anatomy and Physiology*, 8th edn, Hoboken, NJ, John Wiley and Sons Inc.

4 Cardiac Catheterisation

WHAT IS CARDIAC CATHETERISATION?

Cardiac catheterisation is a generic term that refers to a variety of procedures that are used to identify coronary artery disease, abnormalities of heart muscle (infarction or cardiomyopathy), abnormalities of the heart's valves and congenital heart abnormalities (11). These procedures include angiography, ventriculography and right or left catheterisation. As these procedures are invasive, they are carried out in a sterile fluoroscopy suite, also referred to as a catheterisation laboratory (cath lab) (14).

Although, in adults, cardiac catheterisation is most commonly used to diagnose coronary artery disease and assess suitability for revascularisation (11), it is also recommended:

- for patients with suspected restenosis of a prior percutaneous coronary intervention (PCI) and/or stent within the past 9 months;
- prior to cardiac surgery;
- that as cardiac transplant recipients are asymptomatic of atherosclerosis, they should have an angiogram annually;
- to establish whether patients with intractable arrhythmias have coronary artery disease prior to electrophysiological testing;
- for patients with cardiomyopathy in order to identify whether coronary artery disease is the cause of symptoms and evaluate left-ventricular dysfunction;
- to obtain a myocardial biopsy to detect myocarditis;
- to help to differentiate between myocardial restriction and pericardial constriction;
- to assess the extent of valvular regurgitation;
- to obtain haemodynamic information, such as shunt size or pulmonary vascular resistance, in patients with congenital heart disease;
- to evaluate the cardiovascular response to pharmacological intervention (4; 18).

WHAT IS A CORONARY ANGIOGRAM/ARTERIOGRAM?

Coronary angiogram can also be referred to as coronary arteriogram. This procedure is used both to establish whether a patient has significant coronary artery disease and for making treatment decisions about whether to use medical therapy, angioplasty or coronary artery bypass graft (CABG) surgery (9).

For this procedure, a small, hollow tube (catheter) is advanced through the arterial system under fluoroscopy until it reaches the ostium (start) of the coronary artery. Then, contrast dye is injected directly into the coronary artery through the catheter. As the dye flows through the artery, the lumen of the artery can be visualised under fluoroscopy. This shows the outline of the artery and any blockages or narrowings that may exist. In patients who have undergone previous coronary artery bypass surgery, the contrast dye can be injected into the saphenous vein bypass grafts or internal mammary arteries in a similar manner (14).

INTRAVASCULAR ULTRASOUND STUDIES (IVUS)

Coronary angiography is limited, as it can only show a silhouette of the lesion and how it affects the lumen of the coronary artery. It reveals little else about the atherosclerotic plaque or the disease process itself. Using specialised catheters, with transducers mounted cylindrically around the end of the catheter, the cardiologist is able to obtain ultrasound images within the artery, which is referred to as intravascular ultrasound studies (IVUS) (20).

IVUS are capable of providing cross-sectional images of the coronary arteries so that the cardiologists can assess all three layers of the coronary artery, measure the vessel diameter and identify the composition of the plaque causing the atherosclerotic lesion, and whether it is soft, fibrous or calcified (14). This information will help to identify which percutaneous coronary intervention is most appropriate for the patient (18).

VENTRICULOGRAPHY/LEFT AND RIGHT-SIDED CATHETERISATION

A ventriculogram is the injection of contrast dye into the ventricles so that they can be visualised under fluoroscopy. This will assess any reduction in the contractility of the ventricular walls due to stenosed coronary arteries (14). In addition to this, it will help to measure the size of the ventricles, examine the walls of the ventricles and assess the efficiency of the valves in patients with congenital abnormalities, valvular problems, coronary artery disease and cardiomyopathy (1). Injecting large volumes of contrast dye may make the patient feel flushed or experience a temporary hot flush (14).

The catheter used to deliver the contrast dye for a ventriculogram can also measure pressures within the heart structure. These measurements are referred to as left and right catheterisation (9).

Ventriculography may be performed before or after the coronary angiogram. However, coronary angiography is routinely performed first because ventricular function can be obtained through non-invasive methods if complications occur that terminate the study prematurely. In addition, ventriculography may be omitted in patients for whom post-procedural hypotension is anticipated (11).

LEFT VENTRICULOGRAM

The left ventriculogram is an integral part of every coronary catheterisation study (11). A catheter is advanced through the arterial system under fluoroscopy until it reaches the aortic valve. The catheter can then be manipulated across the valve and into the left ventricle (9). The contrast dye is injected rapidly, and an image of the left ventricle cavity is recorded on film as the ventricle contracts. Left-ventricular ejection fraction, namely the percentage of blood present in the left ventricle during diastole that is ejected during systole, can be calculated from the film images (14). The motion of the walls of the left ventricle can be observed and measured. Abnormal wall motion indicates the presence of coronary ischaemia, infarction, aneurysm or hypertrophy (11). In addition, the competence of the mitral valve also may be evaluated during ventriculography. In patients with mitral regurgitation, dye is observed being ejected during systole into the left atrium through an incompetent mitral valve (14).

In addition to visualising the left ventricle, the intracardiac or intravascular pressure in the valves of the left side of the heart can be measured. If either the mitral or the aortic valve is stenosed, the pressures required to eject blood forward are higher than normal because of the small valve orifice (14). Alternatively, these pressures can also be measured by echocardiography (9).

Indications for left ventriculography include:

- identification of left-ventricular function for patients with coronary artery disease, cardiomyopathy or valvular heart disease;
- identification of ventricular septal defects;
- to measure the presence and severity of mitral regurgitation;
- to measure the mass of myocardium for regression of hypertrophy or other similar research studies (11).

CONTRAINDICATIONS TO LEFT VENTRICULOGRAM

To visualise the left ventricle clearly under fluoroscopy requires the rapid injection of 30–40 ml of contrast dye, under high pressure for about 3–4 seconds. The osmolarity and vasodilatation effects of a bolus injection of contrast dye can be poorly tolerated in certain patients. Those identified at high risk of complications during left ventriculography include patients with:

- severe symptomatic aortic stenosis;
- severe congestive heart failure or angina at rest;
- left ventricular thrombus, especially if mobile or protruding into the left ventricle cavity;
- left-sided endocarditis (18).

RIGHT-HEART CATHETERISATION

Right-heart catheterisation is performed to measure intracardiac and intravascular pressures in structures of the right side of the heart. A catheter is inserted through the venous system and advanced into the right atrium, through the tricuspid valve to the right ventricle, thence to the pulmonary artery and finally wedged in a distal pulmonary artery. Pressures are recorded from the vena cava, right atrium, right ventricle, pulmonary artery and pulmonary capillary wedge position (9; 14).

In addition to this, blood samples may be drawn from each chamber as the catheter is advanced, and the amount of oxygen present in each blood sample is measured. Because the right side of the heart normally contains venous blood, a significant increase in the amount of oxygen present in a blood sample may indicate abnormalities, such as:

- when the oxygen saturation in the left pulmonary artery is greater than the oxygen saturation in the right ventricle, this indicates a *persistent ductus arteriosus*;
- when the oxygen saturation in the right ventricle and pulmonary artery is greater than the oxygen saturation in the right atrium, this indicates *ventricular septal defect*;
- when the oxygen saturation in the right atrium exceeds the oxygen saturation in the superior and inferior vena cava, this indicates *atrial septal defect* (9).

However, in modern clinical practice, left-to-right shunts and all forms of valvular heart disease are usually diagnosed by echocardiography without the need for invasive investigation to establish a diagnosis (9).

Cardiac output (the amount of blood pumped by the heart in 1 minute) may be measured during right-heart catheterisation using the thermodilution technique. Because cardiac output can be expected to vary with body size, the term 'cardiac index', which takes height and weight into consideration, is used more often (9, 14).

Indications for right ventriculography are as follows:

- documentation of tricuspid regurgitation;
- assessment of right-ventricle dysplasia for arrhythmias;
- assessment for pulmonary stenosis;
- assessment of abnormalities of pulmonary outflow tract;
- assessment of right-to-left ventricular shunts (11).

COMPLICATIONS OF RIGHT-SIDED HEART CATHETERISATION

The most common problem during right-sided heart catheterisation is arrhythmias from stimulation of the right-ventricular outflow tract, which may result in atrioventricular block or, rarely, right bundle branch block. The majority of these arrhythmias are transient and do not require treatment. However, patients with known left bundle branch block may require a temporary pacemaker if right bundle branch block occurs during right-sided heart catheterisation (11).

AORTOGRAM

An aortogram is when a large volume of contrast dye is rapidly injected under high pressure into the aorta (18). A catheter is advanced through the arterial system under fluoroscopy until it reaches the aortic valve. It is positioned just above the aortic valve but not close enough to interfere with the valve's opening or closing (11).

The indications for an aortogram include:

- aortic regurgitation: the appearance of contrast in the left ventricle during supravalvular aortography confirms the diagnosis;
- to identify coronary artery bypass grafts: when location or number of bypass grafts is not known, a large volume of contrast in the aorta will help to identify them;
- aortic dissection: aortography can accurately identify aortic dissection, showing an intimal flap, an outline of the false lumen and deformity of the true lumen;
- aortic coarctation: aortography enables the measurement of the narrowing of the aorta;
- aortic-to-pulmonary artery communication: the appearance of contrast in the pulmonary artery would aid this diagnosis;
- aortic-to-right-side heart communication (e.g. sinus or Valsalva fistula): the appearance of contrast in the right ventricle whilst the aortic valve is closed would aid this diagnosis;
- aortic aneurysm;
- supravalvular aortic stenosis;
- brachiocephalic or arch vessel disease;
- arterial inflammatory disease (11; 18).

Patients who could not tolerate the rapid injection of a high volume of contrast dye would not be suitable for aortogram. Fortunately, a number of non-invasive techniques are now available, which include transthoracic echocardiogram, transoesophageal echocardiogram, contrast computer tomography (CT) and magnetic resonance imaging (MRI) (11; 18).

CONTRAINDICATIONS TO CARDIAC CATHETERISATION

There are no absolute contraindications for coronary catheterisation. Relative contraindications include:

- unexplained fever, untreated infection;
- severe anaemia with haemoglobin of less than 8 g/dl;

- anticoagulation: international normalised ratio (INR) should be less than 2;
- severe active bleeding;
- acute gastrointestinal bleeding;
- severe electrolyte imbalance (especially hyperkalaemia, as this predisposes to arrhythmias);
- uncontrolled hypertension;
- digitalis toxicity;
- previous contrast allergy but no pretreatment with corticosteroids;
- recent stroke (within a month);
- pregnancy;
- severe renal insufficiency or anuria, unless dialysis is planned after the procedure;
- uncontrolled congestive heart failure;
- active endocarditic or other systemic illness needing stabilisation (4; 11; 24).

COMPLICATIONS

There is a very low mortality and morbidity associated with cardiac catheterisation. Analysis of complications in more than 200,000 patients indicated that the risk of death was less than 0.1%, myocardial infarction less than 0.05%, stroke less than 0.07%, serious ventricular arrhythmia less than 0.5% and major vascular complication (thrombosis, bleeding requiring a transfusion, pseudoaneurysm) less than 1% (1; 11).

WHAT A PATIENT CAN EXPECT WHEN UNDERGOING CARDIAC CATHETERISATION

PRIOR TO THE PROCEDURE

The majority of cardiac catheterisations are performed electively as a day-case procedure; therefore, if a patient is not prepared either psychologically or physically, the procedure should be postponed (11). On arrival to the ward, the nurse will take the patient's biographical details and past medical history and allergy status. If any issues arise from this that might affect the procedure, the nurse should inform the doctor who is performing the procedure. The nurse will take the patient's baseline observations, such as electrocardiogram (ECG), blood pressure, pulse, temperature and blood glucose if the patient is diabetic (4). The nurse should check that the patient has shaved appropriately. A patient identity band, a pair of modesty (paper) pants and a theatre gown will be provided and the patient will be asked to change into them for the procedure (24).

Metformin is contraindicated with intravascular contrast agents; therefore, the nurse should confirm that diabetic patients have stopped taking their metformin at least 24 hours prior to the procedure (14; 20). Anticoagulants such as warfarin should be withheld for several days prior to the procedure. Patients at increased risk of systemic thromboembolism on withdrawal of warfarin, such as those with mitral valve disease or a prior history of systemic thromboembolism, may be admitted to hospital for a few days prior to the procedure to be anticoagulated with heparin while the warfarin is stopped (4). On the day of the procedure, a blood sample should be sent to check that the patient's INR is less than 2, because if the patient's anticoagulation status is higher than that, it increases their risk of bleeding (4). If the patient is on intravenous unfractionated heparin, it may be stopped 4 hours prior to the procedure (22). Alternatively, depending on the cardiologist's preference, this can be continued until the patient's arrival in the cath lab. The activated clotting time (ACT) can then be measured, which will help in calculating how much bolus of intravenous heparin will need to be administered for the procedure (15).

The nurse can inform the patient and their family about the procedure and what to expect and answer any questions that they may have. But it is the cardiologist responsible for the procedure who should obtain written consent from the patient after fully explaining the procedure, including its risks and benefits (4). If the patient is a female of child-bearing age, she will be asked to confirm that she is not pregnant (11). Radiation from x-ray is contraindicated in pregnancy, as it increases the risk of fetal central nerve damage, growth retardation, malformation or miscarriage. As direct irradiation of the uterus can usually be avoided in procedures that involve structures above the diaphragm, cardiac catheterisation and interventions can be justified in an emergency. Extra precautions will be taken during fluoroscopy (1).

Anxiety may provoke angina before the start of the procedure, or the patient may drop their blood pressure and feel faint on arrival in the cath lab (20). Therefore, depending on the hospital protocol, the patient may receive a mild sedative prior to the procedure (14). The nurse should ensure that the written consent has been obtained prior to administering it. Oral diazepam of 5–20 mg can be given to adults orally 1–2 hours prior to the procedure, or diazemuls may be given intravenously just prior to the procedure (20).

Patients should be fasted as per hospital protocol. Prior to any elective surgery, patients are usually fasted to reduce anaesthetic/sedation-induced pulmonary aspiration. In general, clear fluids are allowed up to 2 hours before anaesthesia and light meals up to 6 hours (19). The American Society of Anaesthesiologists recommends that a patient undergoing local analgesia procedures such as cardiac catheterisation should have the same restrictions as those undergoing general anaesthesia. These guidelines are arbitrary and based upon a consensus opinion (19). As prolonged fasting increases patient discomfort, resulting in thirst, nausea, headache, hypoglycaemia, feeling faint and dizziness, the hospital protocol may not follow these guidelines, especially as the risk of the patient needing emergency surgery as a result of cardiac catheterisation is very low (19; 20). As the contrast dye used in the procedure is nephrotoxic, patients with an increased risk, such as those with renal impairment or low cardiac output, should be started on intravenous fluids prior to the procedure if they are fasting (14).

DURING THE PROCEDURE

Once the patient arrives in the cath lab, they will be asked to lie down on the catheterisation table. Electrode stickers will be placed on their torso so that the ECG can monitor their heart rate and rhythm throughout the procedure (11). A probe may be placed on the patient's finger to monitor their blood oxygen saturations and their blood pressure will be monitored intravascularly throughout the procedure. Unless it is against the patient's religious beliefs, the staff will ensure that the proposed access area has been shaved properly; then, the patient will be covered with sterile drapes (11).

Access to the arterial system may be via the femoral, brachial or radial artery (see Chapter 1) (9). However, the most common vascular access site is the femoral approach (11), so this will be the method described here.

Once the patient is lying on the table, both inguinal areas of the thighs will be liberally cleaned with an antiseptic solution. Then, the patient will be covered with sterile cloth, leaving the femoral artery uncovered. Once the preparations to make the patient sterile are completed, a liberal amount of local anaesthetic will be injected (14). The patient should be warned that they may experience some burning as the anaesthetic is being injected (1).

Once the area is anaesthetised, an introducer sheath is inserted into the femoral artery. The patient may feel some tugging and pushing around this time. Usually, there is a small spurt of blood out initially, which shows the physician that the sheath is in the artery (14). The introducer sheath has a one-way valve system which allows the doctor to insert the guidewires and angiogram catheters. This minimises bleeding at the puncture site and avoids stabbing the artery every time a catheter needs to be inserted (14). Although most patients experience little or no discomfort during the procedure, patients should be advised to let staff know if the local anaesthetic begins to wear off so that more may be administered (24). Patients should also be advised to let the staff know if they are experiencing any angina or chest pain so that suitable analgesia can be administered (24).

Once the doctor has the catheter in the appropriate position, the contrast dye is injected. Multiple views are taken of both coronary arteries from different angles to ensure that all proximal segments of the arteries are adequately visualised. For each view, 5–10 ml of contrast dye is injected by hand and a recording of each view is obtained (9). The angles that the pictures are taken at are usually 30°, known as left anterior oblique, and 60°, known as right anterior oblique views. Looking at the coronary artery from these angles provides the physician with the best views to measure and assess a lesion in the coronary arteries. A 'freeze frame' of each view is usually taken so that a hard copy can be placed in the patient's notes (14). Prior to injecting the large volume of contrast dye during the ventriculography or the aortography, the patient should be warned that they may experience a temporary hot flash or flushing while dye is being injected. Some people get embarrassed, as they feel that they have wet themselves, so they should be reassured that they have not (14).

In order to get a better view, the patient may be asked to cough or stop breathing, without bearing down, for a short period of time during the procedure (24). With deep inspiration, the diaphragm descends, preventing it from obstructing the view of the coronary arteries in some radiographic projections. Bearing down (the Valsalva manoeuvre) increases intra-abdominal pressure and may raise the diaphragm, obstructing the view. After the injection of contrast dye, coughing will be requested to help clear the material from the coronary arteries. The rapid movement of the diaphragm also acts as a mechanical stimulant to the heart and helps to prevent bradycardia that may accompany the injection of the contrast dye (24).

As intravenous heparin is no longer required during routine coronary angiography, the femoral sheath is usually removed at the end of the procedure (see Chapter 3) (4).

POST PROCEDURE

Once the procedure is completed, the patient will be escorted back to the ward. On warding, the patient will be attached to a cardiac monitor and blood pressure cuff so that the nurse can obtain their baseline observations. The nurse will check their puncture site, to observe any bleeding, check the pedal pulse and the peripheral skin colour and temperature of the limb below the puncture site (24).

Whilst on bed rest, the nurse should observe the access site every half-hour for signs of bleeding, swelling or haematoma formation (14). Patients should be advised to keep their leg straight, and press over the puncture site before coughing or sneezing. They should inform nursing staff if they feel any blood, wetness or stickiness (3). As tachycardia and a hypotension can indicate that the patient is losing blood, which may not be visible if it is a retroperitoneal bleed, the heart rate and blood pressure should be recorded half-hourly. Often, a patient complaining of low backache is the first symptom of a retroperitoneal bleed (14).

The patient should be allowed to eat and drink immediately after the procedure. Patients should be encouraged to drink plenty of fluid following the procedure in order to compensate for the diuretic action of the contrast dye, as well as to flush out the myocardial and vascular depressant drugs in their system, and to prevent hypotension. If the patient is unable to drink, intravenous fluids should be administered (1).

Patients should remain on bed rest as per hospital protocol. However, one study, by Tagney and Lackie (2005), found that protocols for bed rest following cardiac catheterisation varied in different centres across the United Kingdom. The shortest bed-rest time was 1 hour, whilst the longest was 6 hours. They recommend that once the femoral sheath has been removed after cardiac catheterisation, the patient should lie flat for 1 hour and sit up for 2 hours at 45° before being allowed to mobilise (21).

Once the patient has mobilised and been observed for 30–60 minutes, without any complications, they can be discharged on the same day as the procedure. The doctor should explain the results of the procedure to the patient and a plan of action prior to discharge (24).

Diabetic patients should be advised to omit their metformin for 48 hours after cardiac catheterisation (5). As metformin should only be restarted after the renal function has been re-evaluated and found to be normal, the patient should ask their family doctor to check their urea and electrolytes (15).

As the majority of cardiac catheterisations are performed as day cases, it is advisable for the patient to organise for a responsible adult to drive them home and stay with them until the following morning. If this is not possible, the patient may have to stay overnight in the hospital. In order to protect the haemostasis of the puncture site, patients should be advised to wait until the day after the procedure before they shower (24).

DISCHARGE ADVICE

In order to protect the puncture site from bleeding, patients should be advised:

1. To feel the puncture site for signs of a growing lump over the next 2–3 days. If one develops or they get pins and needles in that leg, they should come back to their local hospital to have it scanned.
2. That they may get a bruise around the puncture site and normally this gets bigger as gravity pulls it down the leg. Unless it is painful, they should not worry about this.
3. That there may be a little bit of blood staining on their underwear. If the blood is bright red and spurting, they should send for an ambulance. Whilst waiting for the ambulance, they should lie down on a firm surface and press firmly just above the puncture site.
4. Although it is very rare for problems like these to occur but in order to minimise them, they should:
   - shower in preference to bathing for the next 2–3 days; if they only have a bath, they should use tepid water;
   - not scrub vigorously over the puncture site;
   - avoid heavy lifting and pulling for the next 2–3 days (24);
   - avoid driving for a week – the DVLA (2006) has no specific recommendations following a cardiac catheterisation. Therefore it is recommended to follow the guidelines for an elective coronary angioplasty which is to avoid driving for a week. All patients with angina have to cease driving if they get symptoms at rest or at the wheel. Group 1 drivers may recommence driving once satisfactory symptom control is achieved. Group 2 drivers with angina have to be free of symptoms for at least 6 weeks, provided that the exercise/functional-test requirement can be met and there are no other disqualifying conditions (7).

CARE PLANS

NURSING CONSIDERATION BEFORE THE PROCEDURE

The principle preparations for cardiac catheterisation are the same as those for any surgical procedure. The primary aim of nursing care is, therefore, to maximise patient safety and comfort during the procedure and optimise conditions for a successful outcome. This is achieved by ensuring that the patient is physically and psychologically prepared for the procedure, and that all documentation, including laboratory results and reports, are available to the cath lab staff (6).

PRE-PROCEDURE CARE PLAN FOR PATIENTS UNDERGOING A CARDIAC CATHETERISATION

Action	Rationale
Obtain a brief history and check that biographical details and next of kin are correct	Checking the patient's biographical details and next of kin ensures that medical records are up-to-date and that in the event of an emergency, the correct person is contacted. Record keeping is a fundamental part of nursing care, ensuring high standards of clinical care and improving communication and dissemination of information (16)
Explain to the patient and their family what a coronary angiogram is and what will happen during and after the procedure. Provide an information booklet about the procedure	The period before coronary catheterisation may be a time of anxiety and fear, for various reasons. Discussion and reassurance may help to relieve some of these feelings (8)
Check whether the patient is allergic to any food, drugs or other substances. Inform the doctor if the patient is allergic to any potential drugs used in the procedure	Patients with a history of allergy to iodine-containing substances, such as seafood or contrast agents, should be given an antihistamine and steroids before the procedure (24). In addition to this, a non-ionic contrast dye may be used for the procedure (4)
Check the medication regime. Metformin should be stopped 24 hours before the procedure	Metformin-associated lactic acidosis can be precipitated by the contrast dye used during the procedure. Although, in patients without renal

Action	Rationale
	failure, metformin can be used up to the day of contrast administration, ideally, it should be avoided 24 hours prior to the procedure (5; 20)
Nephrotoxic drugs and non-steroidal anti-inflammatory drugs should be avoided for a few days prior to the procedure	High doses of contrast dye may cause contrast-induced nephropathy. In order to minimise renal complications, it is advisable to avoid nephrotoxic drugs and non-steroidal anti-inflammatory drugs for several days prior to the procedure (5)
Warfarin should be stopped at least 48 hours prior to the procedure	Warfarin should be withheld for at least 48 hours prior to the procedure, to ensure an INR of less than 2. Patients at high risk of thromboembolism should be admitted for heparinisation while the effects of oral anticoagulation wane (4)
Ideally, the INR should be less than 2 (inform the cardiologist if it is higher)	Warfarin interferes with blood coagulation by blocking the effect of vitamin K. It has a long-acting half-life of 36–42 hours. The anticoagulation effect is described in a measurement of the INR. Therefore, any INR measurement of more than 2 increases the patient's risk of bleeding uncontrollably during and/or after the procedure (2)
If the patient is on low-molecular-weight heparin, the last injection should be given at least 12 hours prior to the procedure	The half-life of a low-molecular-weight heparin administered subcutaneously is about 4 hours (2). Therefore, if prescribed, the morning dose should be omitted prior to the procedure in order to reduce the risk of bleeding (15)
Check that a recent full blood count, and urea and electrolyte blood results are available	Severe anaemia (Hb < 8) and/or severe electrolyte imbalance are contraindicators for cardiac catheterisation (4; 11). The

Action	Rationale
	cause of anaemia should be identified and treated prior to the procedure (11). Low potassium results in increased sensitivity and excitability of the myocardium, which may predispose to arrhythmias (11; 14). Elevation in serum creatinine may indicate problems with kidney function (14). As patients with renal failure have an increased risk of developing contrast nephropathy, risks versus benefits must be considered, and the patient should be hydrated during and after the procedure (1; 5)
Record ECG, blood pressure, pulse, temperature and blood glucose	This information should be evaluated to ensure that the patient is suitable for the procedure (4). It is also used to act as a baseline to compare the patient's vital signs with after the procedure (24)
Cannulate the patient	To provide intravenous access to administer prescribed drugs (14; 24)
Check for patent left and right pedal pulse	This information will be used for comparison in evaluating peripheral pulses after the catheterisation procedure (24)
If it is not against the patient's religious beliefs, ensure that the patient has shaved their groin appropriately	Body hair is removed in order to reduce infection risk during catheterisation (11; 24). Although most catheterisations are usually performed from the right femoral artery, it is expedient to routinely prepare both groins in case of difficulties in catheter advancement which may force a switch to the other groin once the procedure has begun (1)
Record the patient's height and weight	The amount of some of the drugs prescribed during the procedure may

Action	Rationale
	be calculated on the patient's body weight (1; 24)
The patient should be advised of the hospital's pre-procedure fasting protocol	Gastric emptying of water and non-caloric fluids has an average half-time of 10 minutes. Gastric emptying of solids depends on the caloric density of the meal; therefore, patients are usually advised to have a light meal before they start fasting (19)
Patients may wear dentures, glasses and hearing aids during the procedure	Patients are better able to communicate when dentures and hearing aids are in place. Glasses allow the patient to view the procedure better and help to keep the patient oriented to the surroundings (11; 24)
Allow patients to empty their bladder before the procedure	To help make them more comfortable (24)
Ensure that the informed consent has been signed prior to the procedure	This is a legal requirement (15)
If the patient is a female of child-bearing age, she may be asked by the radiographer to sign a form indicating her pregnancy status	Pregnancy is a relative contraindicator in cardiac catheterisation procedures (11). However, as direct irradiation of the uterus can usually be avoided in procedures that involve structures above the diaphragm, fluoroscopic procedures on pregnant women may be justifiable in an emergency situation (1)

POST-PROCEDURE CARE PLAN

Goal/aim of care

The nursing care of patients following cardiac catheterisation is directed towards the prevention and detection of complications (24).

Action	Rationale
On warding, attach the patient to a cardiac monitor and check pulse and blood pressure	In order to observe the patient's vital signs post procedure (14)
Monitoring the pulse	Tachycardia (100–120 beats per minute) is not unusual after catheterisation. This may be a sign of anxiety, an indication of fluid loss due to diuresis or a reaction to medication used during the procedure, such as atropine. Fluids, time and reassurance often bring the heart rate down to more normal levels. Heart rates above 120 beats per minute should be evaluated for other causes, such as haemorrhage, more severe fluid imbalance, fever or arrhythmias (14). If not on betablockers, a bradycardia may indicate a vasovagal response, arrhythmias or an infarction and should be assessed by an ECG and correlated with other clinical signs, such as pain and blood pressure (24)
Blood pressure	Patients may return to the ward with a low blood pressure caused by drugs, such as vasodilators, administered during the procedure. In addition, the contrast dye acts as an osmotic diuretic and patients may become hypotensive due to volume depletion. Patients are thus kept on bed rest until fluid balance is restored, with oral liquids or by intravenous replacement. If the blood pressure is less than 75–80% of baseline, other causes such as blood loss or arrhythmias must be considered and assessed, and the doctor notified (24)

Action	Rationale
Pedal pulse	The most frequent complication of percutaneous procedures is arterial thrombosis. The puncture site in the groin should be checked for visible bleeding, swelling or tenderness. The arterial pulse at the site and at points distal to it should be compared with pulses on the opposite limb and those recorded before the procedure. Capillary filling and the warmth of the limb should also be evaluated. Blanching, cramping, coolness, pain, numbness or tingling may indicate reduced perfusion and must be carefully evaluated. A diminished or absent pulse is a sign of serious arterial occlusion (11; 24). If a compression device is being used to achieve haemostasis, the pressure should be reduced. If this does not improve circulation, medical staff should be informed (24)
Check the puncture site for signs of bleeding or haematoma	Research shows that the majority of bleeding/haematoma was detected by nurses checking the groin (3)
Until the patient is mobile, check these observations half-hourly and ask the patient to report any feelings of wetness, stickiness, warmth or bleeding in the puncture-site area	Research shows that a large proportion of puncture-site bleeding was detected through the patient's calling for assistance (3)
Advise the patient to keep the affected leg straight whilst on bed rest	Bleeding and haematoma formation may occur when a patient moves the limb too vigorously (24)
If the patient is a diabetic, check their blood sugar on warding	To ensure that the patient is not hypoglycaemic, as they may have fasted for long periods prior to the procedure (24)
Ensure that any intravenous pumps are running at the correct rate, and administer any drugs prescribed post procedure	It is the ward nurses' responsibility to ensure that the prescribed drugs, intravenous or oral, are administered correctly (14; 17)

Action	Rationale
Encourage the patient to drink and provide something to eat	Patients are often tired, hungry and uncomfortable when they return from the laboratory (24). Patients should be encouraged to drink plenty in order to prevent hypotension (1)
Observe urine output, as a poor urine output may be the first indication of contrast-induced renal failure	Contrast nephropathy is a recognised complication of coronary angiography (5) and a poor urine output is an early indication of this condition (11). However, as the contrast dye acts as an osmotic diuretic, patients may have an increase in urine output for a short time after the procedure (24)
If a vascular closure device was used to achieve haemostasis, such as an AngioSeal, please follow the manufacturer's guidelines about bed rest and mobilising the patient	Although these devices have been shown to reduce the time taken to obtain haemostasis (1; 11; 23), the patient maintains the risk of developing cardiac complications such as bradycardia or hypotension as a result of the drugs used during the procedure (24); therefore, it is good policy to maintain cardiac monitoring whilst they are on bed rest (13)
If the patient has the femoral sheaths in situ, the cardiologists will advise when the sheaths should be removed	Femoral sheaths are normally removed at the end of cardiac catheterisation, unless heparin was used during the procedure (4)
Once the femoral sheath has been removed and haemostasis has been achieved, the patient must lie flat for 1 hour and then may sit up for 2 hours, or per hospital protocol	Patients are advised to remain on bed rest in order not to disturb the newly formed clot over the puncture site (10). Bed-rest post-sheath removal guidelines vary from hospital to hospital (21)
Once mobile, observations may cease, unless the patient complains of numbness, pins and needles or a lump in the groin area, or the puncture site begins to bleed	Complications such as bleeding or haematomas are normally observed within 10 minutes of ambulation (12)

Action	Rationale
Advise patients to press on the puncture site if they cough or sneeze, and to inform the nurse if they experience any chest pain	Patients are advised to press on the puncture site while coughing or sneezing in order to prevent the newly formed clot from being disturbed. Chest pain may indicate potential cardiac complications; therefore, nurses should be aware of it if it is present (3; 24)
Prior to discharge, the patient should be instructed about puncture-site care, and informed of any signs and symptoms which require a doctor's review. A discharge leaflet should be provided	So that patients will be aware of potential complications post discharge and know what to do in the event of these occurring (11)
Any changes in medication should be discussed with the patient	When discharging a patient, it is the nurses' responsibility to inform the patient about the medication that they have been prescribed so that they will take it correctly at home (17)
If the patient normally takes metformin, they should be advised to have their urea and electrolytes checked by their family doctor 48 hours after the procedure and restart it when advised to do so by them	Metformin is contraindicated in patients with renal dysfunction, as determined by elevated serum creatinine levels. Therefore, metformin should only be resumed after the renal function is found to be normal (15)

REFERENCES

1. Baim, D. S. (2006) *Grossman's Cardiac Catheterisation: Angiography and Intervention*, 7th edn, Philadelphia, PA, Lippincott Williams & Wilkins.
2. Blann, A., Landray, M. and Lip, G. (2002) 'An overview of antithrombotic therapy', *British Medical Journal*, **325**: 762–5.
3. Botti, M., Williamson, B. and Steen, K. (2001) 'Coronary angiography observations: Evidence-based or ritualistic practice?', *Heart & Lung: The Journal of Acute and Critical Care*, **30**(2): 138–45.
4. Braunweld, E., Zipes, D. and Libby, P. (2001) *Heart Disease: A Textbook of Cardiovascular Medicine*, Vol. 1, 6th edn, London, W.B. Saunders Co.
5. Brinker, J. A., Davidson, C. J. and Laskey, W. (2005) 'Preventing in-hospital cardiac and renal complications in high-risk PCI patients', *European Heart Journal Supplements*, **7** (Suppl G): G13–25, available online at *www.eurheartj/sui054*.

6. Carter, L. and Lamerton, M. (1996) 'Understanding balloon mitral valvuloplasty: The Inoue technique', *Intensive and Critical Care Nursing*, **12**: 147–54.

7. DVLA (2006) *For Medical Practitioners: At a Glance Guide to the Current Medical Standards of Fitness to Drive*, February, available online at *www.dvla.gov.uk*.

8. Hughes, S. (2002) 'The effects of pre-operative information', *Nursing Standard*, **16**: 28, 33–7.

9. Julian, D. G., Cowan, J. C. and McLenachan, J. M. (2005) *Cardiology*, 8th edn, London, Elsevier Saunders.

10. Keeling, A., Fisher, C., Haugh, K., Powers, E. and Turner, M. (2000) 'Reducing time in bed after percutaneous transluminal coronary angioplasty (TIBS III)', *American Journal of Critical Care*, **9**(3): 185–7.

11. Kern, M. (2003) *The Cardiac Catheterisation Handbook*, 4th edn, London, Mosby.

12. Logemann, T., Luetmer, P., Kaliebe, J., Olson, K. and Murdock, D. (1999) 'Two versus six hours of bed rest following left-sided cardiac catheterisation and a meta-analysis of early ambulation trials', *The American Journal of Cardiology*, **84**: 486–8.

13. Montalsecot, G., Andersen, H., Antoniucer, D., Betriu, A., de Boer, M., Grip, L., *et al.* (2004) 'Recommendations on percutaneous coronary intervention for the reperfusion of acute ST elevation myocardial infarction', *Heart*, 90, available online at *http://heart.bmjjournals.com/cgi/content/full/90/6/e37*.

14. Morton, P. G., Fontaine, D. K., Hudak, C. M. and Gallo, B. M. (2005) *Critical Care Nursing: A Holistic Approach*, 8th edn, Philadelphia, PA, Lippincott Williams & Wilkins.

15. Norell, M. and Perrins, J. (2003) *Essential Interventional Cardiology*, Philadelphia, PA, W.B. Saunders Co.

16. Nursing Midwifery Council (2002a) *Guidelines for Records and Record Keeping*, London, Nursing and Midwifery Council, April.

17. Nursing Midwifery Council (2002b) *Guidelines for the Administration of Medicines*, London, Nursing and Midwifery Council.

18. Rosendorff, C. (2005) *Essential Cardiology: Principles and Practice*, 2nd edn, Totowa, NJ, Humana Press.

19. Soreide, E., Eriksson, L. I., Hirlekar, G., Eriksson, H., Henneberg, W., Sandin, R., Raeder (Task Force on Scandinavian Pre-operative Fasting Guidelines, Clinical Practice Committee Scandinavian Society of Anaesthesiology and Intensive Care Medicine) (2005) 'Pre-operative fasting guidelines: An update', *Acta Anaesthesiologica Scandinavica*, **49**: 1041–7.

20. Swanton, R. H. (2003) *Pocket Consultant Cardiology*, 5th edn, Oxford, Blackwell Publishing.

21. Tagney, J. and Lackie, D. (2005) 'Bed-rest post femoral arterial sheath removal: What is safe practice? A clinical audit', *Nursing in Critical Care*, **10**(4): 167–73.

22. Thompson, P. (1997) *Coronary Care Manual*, London, Churchill Livingstone.

23. Topol, E. J. (1999) *Textbook of Interventional Cardiology*, 3rd edn, London, W.B. Saunders Co.

24. Woods, S., Froelicher, E. and Motzer, S. (2000) *Cardiac Nursing*, 4th edn, Philadelphia, PA, Lippincott Williams & Wilkins.

5 Percutaneous Coronary Intervention

CORONARY CIRCULATION

The heart is a muscular pump, which receives oxygenated blood through a network of arteries called the coronary arteries (29) (Figure 5.1). There are two major coronary arteries: the right and the left. These arise from the aorta. The right coronary artery runs down the groove between the right atrium and right ventricle. In most hearts, this branch supplies the sinus node, the atrioventricular node and bundle of His, the right ventricle and inferior part of the left ventricle (11). The left coronary artery also arises from the aorta, immediately above the aortic valve. This artery divides into two major branches known as the left anterior descending artery (LAD) and the left circumflex artery (LCX). The LAD passes down the anterior wall of the left ventricle towards the apex of the myocardium, and supplies oxygenated blood to the interventricular septum and the anterior wall of the left ventricle. The circumflex passes around in the groove between the left atria and the left ventricle and supplies the lateral and posterior aspects of the left ventricle (11).

These major arteries traverse the external surface of the myocardium, sending branches perpendicularly into the muscle mass. The arteries divide to form arterioles and capillaries similar to those elsewhere in the body, and the venules and veins join to form larger venous channels. Virtually all the blood from the left coronary artery eventually drains into the coronary sinus; the blood from the right coronary artery drains mainly into anterior cardiac veins. From these veins, the blood passes into the right atrium (1). This is known as the coronary arterial tree.

CORONARY ARTERY DISEASE

Coronary artery disease (CAD) is the commonest cause of heart disease and is, significantly, the most common single cause of death in the affluent countries of the world. In the overwhelming majority of cases, disease of the coronary arteries is due to atherosclerosis (11).

Atherosclerosis is a complex disease. Although the initiating causes of atherosclerosis are not completely understood, it is believed that it is probably caused when fatty substances (especially cholesterol and triglycerides) accumulate in the walls of medium and large arteries. Depending on their location and the

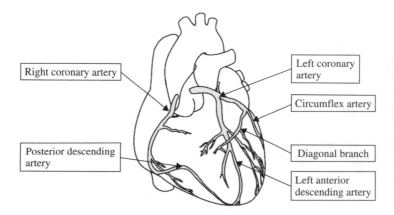

Figure 5.1. The heart and coronary arteries.

presence of relevant risk factors, these fatty substances may develop into the characteristic atherosclerosis lesion – a fibrolipid plaque. Plaques may vary in their composition. At one extreme are soft fatty plaques, containing a large pool of cholesterol and its esters, separated from the lumen of the artery by a thin fibrous cap. The plaque provides a rough surface that causes blood platelets to release the hormone platelet-derived growth factor (PDGF), which promotes the proliferation of smooth muscle fibres. It is not surprising, then, that at the other extreme there are solid plaques, consisting of smooth muscle cells and connective tissue. Calcification may be superimposed (11; 29).

Although the atheromatous plaque may itself narrow the lumen of the artery, it is also prone to fracture. This allows the necrotic core to ulcerate and trigger off platelet aggregation and fibrin deposition. This is a repetitive process and leads to further narrowing, which may proceed to complete occlusion (11).

CAD may present in any of the following ways:

- stable angina;
- unstable angina;
- non-Q-wave myocardial infarction (MI)/non-ST-segment elevated myocardial infarction (NSTEMI);
- ST-segment elevated myocardial infarction (STEMI);
- heart failure;
- sudden death;
- as an incidental finding (symptomatic) (11).

TREATMENT FOR CORONARY ARTERY DISEASE

Until 1977, coronary artery bypass graft surgery (CABG) was the only alternative to medicine for the treatment of CAD. This is a surgical procedure in which a portion of a blood vessel (usually a leg vein or chest wall artery) is grafted onto a coronary artery so as to bypass an obstruction or narrowing in that coronary artery (13; 29). However, the development of the first percutaneous transluminal coronary angioplasty (PTCA), performed by Gruentzig in 1977, marked major innovation in the treatment of CAD (16).

During a PTCA, the narrowed portion of the coronary artery can be enlarged selectively without surgery by the insertion of a long, thin balloon to open the blocked artery (11). When the balloon is inflated, this expands the lumen of the coronary artery by stretching and tearing the atherosclerotic plaque and vessel wall and, to a lesser extent, by redistributing atherosclerotic plaque along its longitudinal axis. There is no evidence that balloon PTCA compresses atherosclerotic plaque (5).

Unfortunately, in about 25–40% of patients who just have PTCA, the artery re-narrows (restenoses) within about 6 months and the angina returns (11). Therefore, new devices were developed in the early 1990s to help to improve the outcome of a PTCA. These devices were designed to act as a scaffold (e.g. stent), to remove (e.g. atherectomy) or ablate (e.g. laser) the atherosclerotic plaque (5). These devices have enabled physicians to non-surgically treat a wide variety of coronary artery problems. Nowadays, as coronary angioplasty encompasses the use of both the inflation of balloons and these devices, they are generically referred to as percutaneous coronary intervention (PCI) (5).

COMPARISON BETWEEN PERCUTANEOUS CORONARY INTERVENTION AND CORONARY ARTERY BYPASS GRAFT SURGERY

The use of PCI as an alternative to CABG surgery in patients with CAD has expanded dramatically over the past two decades (20).

The advantages that a PCI offers over CABG surgery include:

- No general anaesthetic is required.
- Cardiopulmonary bypass machine and its inherent risks are avoided.
- The emotional stress of awaiting dilation is reduced compared with that of awaiting surgery.
- The hospital stay is shorter with PCI; on average, PCI requires a hospital stay of 12–24 hours, whereas CABG requires a stay of 3–7 days.
- Barring complications, the average cost of PCI is substantially lower than that of CABG.
- Patients are able to resume their normal life sooner after a PCI; for example, patients can return to work within 7–10 days after a PCI, whereas patients undergoing a CABG return to work within 6 weeks.
- If a patient has a clotting disorder or has recently had thrombolysis, they can be treated in an emergency with PCI.
- If the PCI is unsuccessful, a CABG can still be performed (whereas a second CABG operation carries a much higher risk).

- Depending on the lesion, some patients who are unfit for CABG might still benefit from a PCI.
- Mortality rates associated with first-time angioplasty and CABG are similar (the PCI mortality rate ranges from 0 to 2%; the CABG mortality rate ranges from 1.5 to 4%) (1; 16).

Despite the above advantages, not all patients with CAD are suitable for PCI, such as patients who have left main stem disease who are less suitable, as are some patients with multi-vessel disease and chronic occlusions. Patient selection is therefore important (1). All patients undergo a coronary angiogram prior to either procedure, which helps to determine which revascularisation technique would be more beneficial to them (11). A PCI is indicated in patients whose coronary arteries have at least a 70% narrowing (16).

PERCUTANEOUS CORONARY INTERVENTIONS

Percutaneous refers to the insertion of a catheter into the body through a small puncture in the skin, usually into an artery, while *coronary* identifies that it is a coronary artery to be dilated, and *intervention* relates to a technique for remodelling a blood vessel through the introduction of a balloon catheter, expandable stent or another specialised tool for treating a diseased artery (13). These specialised tools include laser angioplasty, atherectomy and rotablations.

PERCUTANEOUS TRANSLUMINAL CORONARY ANGIOPLASTY

During balloon angioplasty, access to the coronary vessels is gained via the femoral, radial or brachial artery. A balloon catheter is then passed over a guidewire and into the stenosed (narrowed) segment of the artery. The balloon is then inflated, causing disruption of the stenosis. As a recent cholesterol blockage is usually as soft as margarine, it is easily squashed and plastered to the artery wall, thus clearing the blockage. Therefore, this produces a substantial increase in the diameter of the artery (11) (Figure 5.2).

One of the biggest problems associated with PTCA was that about 25–40% of the dilated arteries tended to re-narrow (restenose), with return of angina within 6 months of the procedure (11). The cause of the restenosis is believed to be an excessive healing response to the balloon dilation. One problem was that the dilated lesion acted as a potential site for platelet adhesion and aggregation; thus, a thrombus could form (16). To reduce this risk, patients are normally given a combination of aspirin and clopidogrel for at least 1 month (11). The other problem was the development of scar tissue over the lesion site, almost like keloid formation following surgery. Since the treated arteries are only 2–3 mm in diameter, there is not much room to accommodate the scar tissue (24). The development of stents has dramatically reduced restenosis; therefore, the majority

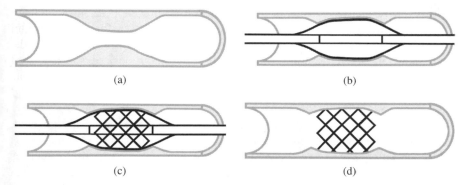

Figure 5.2. (a) Narrowed artery before angioplasty and stent. (b) Balloon inflated to compress plaque. (c) Stent opened up by the inflated balloon. (d) Stent left in position in the artery.

of patients have a coronary artery stent implanted when they undergo a coronary angioplasty. Restenosis can still occur, but the rates are around 10% and are substantially lower than in PTCA without stenting (11).

STENTS

Stents are flexible metal (usually steel) cylindrical structures, usually with a mesh or coil design (1). They are crimped onto the outside of an angioplasty balloon. The balloon-mounted stent is then passed into the dilated segment of the artery and the balloon is inflated. This expands and deploys the stent. The balloon is then deflated and removed, leaving the stent as a permanent internal scaffolding within the artery (11). Nowadays, where appropriate, stents can be deployed without the balloon's predilating the narrowed lumen. This technique is called direct stenting (15).

Coronary artery dissection was a major problem with PTCA. The pressures used to inflate the balloon may cause the normal three-layered arterial wall to crack, and the inner layer of the artery to peel back from the middle layer, thus blocking the lumen of the artery. This would impede blood flow, causing an acute myocardial infarction (AMI) and possibly death. Prior to the advent of stents, emergency CABG surgery was required to save the patient if a dissection occurred. As stents act as a scaffold within the lumen of the coronary artery, they can hold back dissection flaps, thus decreasing the need for emergency CABG surgery and the risk of myocardial infarction (MI) (13). Studies have shown that the introduction of coronary stents reduced the risk of acute complications, thereby lowering the need for emergency CABG surgery to less than 1% and reducing the rate of recurrent symptoms due to restenosis. Because of these results, coronary stents are now used in more than 90% of patients undergoing PCI (20).

However, restenosis is a major short and long-term complication of PCI. As many stents are made of stainless steel, they may act as a focus for thrombi accumulation. Normally, the lining of the coronary artery forms a layer over the metal stent (endothelialisation), thus providing a smooth surface so that blood will not stick to it. Until the stent is endothelialised, it is important that patients take appropriate antiplatelet medication (16).

Research into reducing stent restenosis is ongoing. Making stents from newer alloys or compounds as alternatives to stainless steel are being investigated. Drug-eluting stents have been shown to reduce late recurrence of restenosis (11; 20). Drug-eluting stents are coated with a polymer onto which drugs such as heparin, paclitaxel, actinomycin D or rapamycin are bonded. It is believed that the gradual release of these drugs into the coronary vasculature at the site of the atherosclerotic plaque will inhibit restenosis by limiting smooth muscle cell proliferation and inflammation, thus allowing re-endothelialisation to proceed normally (16).

Although rarely performed nowadays, another technique for reducing restenosis is *brachytherapy*. With this technique, a radioactive ribbon is advanced into the artery after a normal angioplasty or stent procedure. The treated arterial segment is then irradiated with either a beta or a gamma-emitting radiation source. It was found that brachytherapy delays endothelialisation of the stent and leaves the patient at risk of late thrombosis for much longer than after a simple stent procedure. Brachytherapy is generally reserved for patients in whom the lesion has already restenosed once (11).

Long-standing blockages can be very hard and may not be amenable to balloon angioplasty alone. Therefore, alternative techniques have been developed to open these blockages. These include laser angioplasty and atherectomy (11).

LASER

The acronym LASER stands for 'light amplification through stimulated emission of radiation' (16). The laser energy is transmitted through a catheter containing numerous glass fibres. These fibres transmit the light energy to cut through stenotic or occluded lesions (11; 16).

Laser angioplasty is performed much like a standard balloon angioplasty procedure. One difference, though, is that before the laser is activated, everyone in the room (including the patient) must don protective eyewear. The atherosclerotic plaque is vaporised by the laser energy (16).

Stenotic lesions best suited for laser angioplasty include those that are long and diffuse (longer than 15–20 mm), ostial in location, highly calcified and in vein grafts totally occluded. Risks associated with laser angioplasty include perforation of the coronary artery, dissections and aneurysms (16).

CORONARY ATHERECTOMY

Atherectomy is the process of removing atherosclerotic plaque from the coronary artery by cutting or ablating it. Three devices developed for this purpose have been approved for coronary intervention. These are directional coronary atherectomy (DCA), transluminal extraction catheter (TEC) and rotational ablation (Rotablator) (13; 16).

Potential complications of all atherectomy devices include perforation of the coronary artery, abrupt closure embolisation distal to the lesion site and MI. The rate of restenosis and other complications is comparable to that with PTCA (16).

Directional coronary atherectomy (DCA)

Directional coronary atherectomy is performed using a specially designed catheter with a metal cutting chamber that contains a cylindrical cutter. It is positioned so that the opening for the blade faces the lesion. A low-pressure balloon on the opposite side of the catheter is inflated, thus forcing the atherosclerotic plaque into the opening near the cutting blade. The cutting blade turns at approximately 1,200 revolutions per minute (rpm) and is then slowly advanced along the length of the lesion, cutting the plaque and collecting it in the nose cone of the catheter. The procedure is repeated until the atherosclerotic plaque is sufficiently removed. The catheter, laden with plaque, is then withdrawn from the patient (16). Nowadays, stenting has largely replaced DCA (13).

Transluminal extraction catheter (TEC)

The TEC device is a percutaneous, over-the-wire, motor-driven cutting and aspiration system. The TEC device is unique in that it has a detachable vacuum bottle. The cutting device is advanced over the guidewire and positioned 1–2 mm proximal to the stenotic lesion. The cutting blade rotates at 750 rpm and is manually advanced along the length of the stenotic lesion, pulling excised plaque and thrombus through the TEC catheter and into the vacuum bottle. Several passes across the lesion are performed. Adjunctive balloon angioplasty may be performed after use of the TEC (16).

Rotational ablation device

The rotational ablation device, Rotablator, is a high-speed rotating, abrasive, burr-tipped catheter that ablates the atherosclerotic plaque in the coronary artery. The device consists of a football-shaped (olive-shaped) steel burr (1.25–2.5 mm in diameter) that is embedded with microscopic diamond particles in the front half. It is rotated by an external turbine up to speeds of 200,000 rpm. This pulverises the hard atherosclerotic plaque into micro particles that are absorbed into the patient's circulatory system. The burr is advanced through the lesion in a slow and steady manner. After several passes have been performed, it is removed and a decision for a larger burr or complementary balloon inflation is made (13; 16).

The Rotablator has proved to be especially effective in complex stenotic lesions that are calcified, tortuous, small in diameter, ostial or diffuse in character (16).

The complication and restenosis rates are similar to balloon angioplasty. A specific complication of the rotablator is a temporary no-reflow phenomenon with creatine kinase increase in some patients. This problem may necessitate insertion of a prophylactic pacemaker wire, especially for right-coronary lesions (13).

Thrombus aspiration system

A thrombus aspiration system is a device that can suck the blood clot out of the artery. One device – the AngioJet Rheolytic Thrombectomy System – uses high-pressure water jets, which are directed backward into the catheter, which creates a strong suction at the space near the tip and effective thrombus evacuation occurs (13).

The AngioJet System removes the thrombus from the artery as safely as thrombolytic therapy and, in some lesions, reduces the risk of the thrombus's breaking up, resulting in a blockage further down the artery (13).

PRIMARY/RESCUE ANGIOPLASTY

Coronary angioplasty and stenting were reserved for elective procedures initially, and were withheld from patients with acute myocardial infarctions (AMIs) because of concerns over acute stent thrombosis (5). However, with advances in stent deployment, improvements in antiplatelet therapy and increases in operator experience, PCIs are now being performed on more acutely ill patients and two new terms are now being used in the cardiology catheterisation laboratory (cath lab): rescue angioplasty and primary angioplasty.

It has been established that coronary reperfusion can be achieved by emergency PCI. By using a guidewire and balloon catheter, it is technically easier to cross a total occlusion consisting of a fresh thrombus than to cross a long-standing occlusion of a coronary artery (5). Thus, wire-guided balloon angioplasty can be useful to achieve reperfusion in two quite different circumstances. One method is a *rescue angioplasty*. This is when thrombolysis has failed to reperfuse the coronary artery following a STEMI and a PCI is usually performed within 24 hours of the event (5).

Another method is a *primary angioplasty*. This is when an infarct-related coronary artery is dilated during the acute phase of an MI without prior administration of a thrombolytic agent. As primary angioplasty does not have the risk of bleeding associated with thrombolytic therapy, it can be used on patients believed to be at high risk of bleeding complications (such as cardiovascular accident (CVA), prolonged cardiopulmonary resuscitation (CPR), bleeding diathesis, severe hypertension or recent surgery). Patients without these risks can still have thrombolytics, after a primary angioplasty if residual thrombus is observed. Primary angioplasty may offer distinct advantages in reducing the length of hospital stay and eliminating the need for additional intervention in many cases (16).

Like thrombolysis, the sooner the patient receives the primary angioplasty, the more they will benefit from it. Several studies have shown that primary PCI is preferable to intravenous thrombolysis for the treatment of an AMI. They recommend that patients should receive the primary angioplasty within 6 hours of the chest pain (15). Patients undergoing a primary PCI may be attached to an intra-aortic balloon pump (IABP) during the procedure. The prophylactic aortic counter-pulsation created by the IABP can improve overall clinical outcome in patients undergoing a primary PCI (15).

RESTENOSIS AND PHARMACOTHERAPY

When a stent has been deployed in a coronary artery, a process called 'endothe-lialisation' occurs. This is when the endothelial cells of the coronary artery wall grow and cover all the struts of the stent. This takes a period of about 2–4 weeks. At the end of this time, the coronary stent is effectively incorporated into the wall of the artery, with no bare metal exposed to the circulating blood. Until the stent is fully endothelialised, there is a risk that the circulating blood might stick to the bare metal; thus, the stent itself could act as a focus for thrombus formation (11). Therefore, appropriate antiplatelet and antithrombin drugs are an important aspect of reducing stent restenosis.

Improvements in stenting techniques, particularly high-pressure balloon infla-tion, were developed around the same time as the pharmacological management for the prevention of stent thrombosis improved. Thus, with this combination, stent thrombosis now occurs in fewer than 1% of modern PCIs (26). However, research into pharmacotherapy and stent thrombosis continues; therefore, drug regimes may vary from centre to centre. They are usually based on latest research findings and the cardiologist's preference.

Drugs normally administered to prevent stent thrombosis

When blood vessels are damaged or ruptured, the body's natural haemostatic response must be quick, localised to the region and carefully controlled in order to minimise loss of blood. The body has three basic mechanisms to prevent blood loss: vascular spasm, blood coagulation (clotting) and platelet plug forma-tion (29). As performing a PCI will trigger these haemostatic mechanisms both at the site of insertion of the introduction sheath and in the coronary arteries, drugs are given to prevent this.

Coronary vasodilators

Nitrates act as a smooth muscle relaxant, which causes coronary vasodilation without increasing myocardial oxygen consumption; therefore, they may be ad-ministered during a PCI in order to minimise vascular spasm (16).

Heparin

Forming a blood clot is a complex procedure in which coagulation factors activate each other. It results in a gel-like substance, intended to plug the break in the vascular vessel in order to reduce bleeding. Normally, it does not extend beyond the site of the wound into general circulation (29). However, when a blood clot does form in an unbroken vessel, it is called a thrombus. If a thrombus was to lodge in the circulatory system, it would deprive the area distal to it of oxygenated blood. Therefore, it may cause an MI, stroke, pulmonary embolism, renal embolism or peripheral vascular thrombosis (29). In order to minimise this risk, an anticoagulant such as unfractionated heparin (UFH) is usually administered during a PCI, in order to prevent a thrombus's forming at the site of arterial injury or on the coronary guidewire and catheters used during the procedure (15).

Heparin is recommended for patients in whom a prolonged (more than 20 minutes' arterial time) catheterisation procedure is anticipated or in whom prior clinical indications for use of heparin exist (e.g. thrombotic tendency, known severe peripheral vascular disease, embolic phenomenon on previous study) (13).

The amount of heparin administered depends upon the patient's weight and whether GPIIb/IIIa inhibitors are being administered (15). However, an intravenous (5,000 U) bolus dose of unfractionated heparin can achieve therapeutic anticoagulation status in 94% of patients (13). Unlike most drugs, it is impossible to determine the timing of the peak effect of heparin, or when plasma levels of heparin are diminished and the drug has 'worn off' (9). The advantages of UFH are that it has a short half-life and, by monitoring the activated clotting time (ACT), the dose can be titrated during the PCI (20).

Unfractionated heparin works by inhibiting the clotting of blood and the formation of fibrin clots (16). Prior to sheath removal, the patient must have some ability to clot at the arterial puncture site, to prevent serious bleeding complications or prolonged compression of the artery. Thus, the anticoagulant 'effect' of the heparin (not the antiplatelets) must be reduced prior to sheath removal. To date, it has been difficult to determine when the ability to clot has returned to an appropriate level at which it is safe to remove the sheath. Protocols vary, recommending that ACT levels are anywhere between 150 and 200 seconds (9).

Problems associated with measuring ACT prior to sheath removal include variability amongst differing machines on the market, ACT tests lose their reliability below 225 seconds and, finally, many wards do not have access to a machine. To overcome these problems, many centres prefer to wait for 4–6 hours after the PCI to ensure haemostasis rather than risk removing the sheath too soon (9).

Low-molecular-weight heparin (LMWH) has replaced unfractionated heparin for the treatment of patients with NSTEMI or unstable angina. However, it is more difficult to monitor levels of anticoagulation with LMWH during PCI; therefore, empiric dosing has also been developed (20). Thus, a patient can still undergo a PCI even if they have received a dose of LMWH that day.

Bivalirudin

Direct thrombin inhibition has been evaluated as an alternative to heparin during PCI. It has been found that bivalirudin may be particularly useful for patients at high risk of bleeding, such as elderly people or those with renal insufficiency (20). Trials have shown bivalirudin to be more effective than heparin and as effective as heparin with glycoprotein IIb/IIIa in treating unstable angina when undergoing a PCI. Bivalirudin has two other great advantages over heparin. Firstly, it causes significantly less bleeding, particularly at the access site, and, secondly, sheaths can be removed sooner without the need for ACT testing (9).

Bivalirudin is administered as a bolus at the start of the PCI procedure, and maintained with an infusion. Most physicians discontinue bivalirudin at the end of the procedure, although the package insert calls for continuation for 4 hours after the procedure. The half-life of bivalirudin is 25 minutes in patients with normal renal function and longer in patients with renal disease. It takes approximately two half-lives for the drug levels to fall to a non-therapeutic level. Thus, sheaths can be safely removed in most patients 2 hours after bivalirudin has been discontinued (9). However, for patients on dialysis, it may take up to 8 hours before bivalirudin has reached a non-therapeutic level (2). As bivalirudin levels fall quickly and reliably after the drug has been discontinued, it is not necessary to monitor the coagulation of the patient's blood with an ACT (9). However, there is no rapid reversal agent available in the event of a life-threatening bleed (2).

Glycoprotein IIb/IIIa inhibitors

A thrombus may occur within a blood vessel as a result of platelet formation. This may be initiated by a roughened endothelial surface of a blood vessel as a result of atherosclerosis, infection or trauma. These conditions induce adhesion of the platelets; therefore, a blood clot may develop despite anticoagulation and/or fibrinolysis (29).

The glycoprotein (GP) IIb/IIIa receptors on a platelet serve as the 'final common pathway' of platelet aggregation by bridging adjacent platelets together, thus forming a thrombus (20). The GP IIb/IIIa inhibitors block these receptors, preventing the platelets from binding and forming a thrombus. There are three agents currently available: abciximab, tirofiban and eptifibatide. All are given intravenously. They reduce peri-procedural complications such as MI (11); they can be used in all PCI procedures and side effects are rare. In most centres, however, they are used mainly in higher-risk PCI procedures (acute patients, bifurcation lesions, etc.) (11).

Aspirin

Aspirin is an antiplatelet agent. It acts by irreversibly inhibiting the cyclooxygenase, thereby blocking platelet synthesis of thromboxane A_2 – a humeral mediator that promotes platelet aggregation (20). Aspirin exerts its inhibitory effect within 60 minutes of oral administration, and its effect on platelet inhibition lasts for up to 7 days after the last dose of aspirin. The minimum effective aspirin dosage in the setting of PCI has not been established (20). Although trials have not shown that aspirin does reduce angiographic or clinical restenosis, it continues to be administered post PCI because aspirin is known to prevent cardiovascular death, MI and stroke in patients with CAD (20).

Aspirin-intolerant patients. Thienopyridine derivatives or GP IIb/IIIa inhibitors should be substituted for aspirin in patients who are unable to take aspirin because of hypersensitivity or major gastrointestinal intolerance. However, studies have shown that aspirin and a proton pump inhibitor twice a day are safer than clopidogrel in patients with a history of upper gastrointestinal bleed (21). Hypersensitivity to aspirin can be manifested as acute asthma, urticaria, angioedema or, less commonly, as a systemic anaphylactoid reaction (20).

Thienopyridine derivatives (clopidogrel, ticlopidine)

Thienopyridine derivatives (clopidogrel, ticlopidine) are antiplatelet agents. They produce irreversible inhibition of the platelet adenosine diphosphate receptor, thereby weakening platelet aggregation in response to adenosine diphosphate released from activated platelets. The two thienopyridine derivatives used in the trials were ticlopidine and clopidogrel. It was found that clopidogrel and ticlopidine were just as good as each other, but clopidogrel produced fewer side effects and is easier to administer (20).

Aspirin and clopidogrel have complementary mechanisms of action, and the combination of these agents inhibits platelet aggregation to a greater extent than either agent alone. The combination of aspirin and clopidogrel is better than systemic anticoagulation therapy (such as warfarin) for the prevention of complications after coronary stent insertion. Therefore, this combination has become the standard of care for all PCI patients with stents (20).

High loading doses of clopidogrel (600 mg) cause very pronounced platelet inhibition, reaching peak concentration 2 hours after administration and lasting for 2 days. The only concern that exists with regard to the early administration of clopidogrel is in patients who may have to undergo urgent surgery (a rare situation). If required, a platelet transfusion and/or the use of drugs such as aprotinin can be administered to counter the effects of the clopidogrel (15).

Trials for optimum clopidogrel dosage are ongoing; therefore, dosage may vary from centre to centre. Popma *et al.* (20) have reviewed the current data and they recommend that:

- A loading dose of 300 mg of clopidogrel should be administered at least 6 hours prior to planned PCI.
- If clopidogrel is started less than 6 hours prior to planned PCI, a 600-mg loading dose of clopidogrel should be administered.

- In addition to aspirin, the PCI patient should receive clopidogrel (75 mg/d) for at least 9–12 months.
- If ticlopidine is used instead of clopidogrel, a loading dose of 500 mg should be given at least 6 hours before planned PCI. The ticlopidine should be continued for at least 2 weeks after the PCI (20).

One main side effect of ticlopidine is that it may cause neutropenia and thrombocytopenia, thus necessitating blood-count monitoring (20). Although side effects with clopidogrel are rare, they do include diarrhoea, rash, gastrointestinal disturbances, haemorrhage and neutropenia (16).

COMPLICATIONS

As a specialised form of cardiac catheterisation, PCI is attended by the usual risks related to invasive percutaneous cardiac procedures (see Chapter 3). In contrast to diagnostic procedures, the larger-calibre guided catheters used for angioplasty are more likely to result in damage to the proximal coronary artery and cause local bleeding complications at the catheter introduction site (2). Coronary artery dissection and abrupt vessel closure are two major complications associated with PCI, which may result in death or emergency CABG surgery (2). However, improvements in stenting techniques and developments in pharmacotherapy have reduced these complications to 1% (20).

Although the indications for PCI have expanded nowadays to include patients with more severe CAD (i.e. total occlusions, multivessel disease, recent or ongoing MI, poor left ventricular function), the rate of complications associated with PCI has not increased (16).

WHAT A PATIENT CAN EXPECT WHEN UNDERGOING
A PERCUTANEOUS CORONARY INTERVENTION

Prior to the procedure

If the patient is to undergo an elective PCI, they may be invited to attend a pre-admission clinic. Attending pre-admission clinic provides the nursing staff with the opportunity to explain to the patient and their family/carers what an angioplasty entails and what they can expect to happen on the day, and allows opportunities to ask questions, in order to reduce their anxieties (10). In addition to this, the nurse can complete the patient's biographical details and take a medical history and allergy status. If any issues arise from this that might affect the procedure, the medical staff should be advised so that they can address them (5). The patient's height and weight should be recorded. A pre-procedure electrocardiogram (ECG) can be obtained and blood can be taken to test the urea and electrolytes and a full blood count performed. If the patient cannot attend a pre-admission clinic, then the nurse can do this on the day of admission.

Whilst at pre-admission clinic, diabetic patients should be advised to stop their metformin at least 24 hours before the procedure, as it is contraindicated with intravascular contrast dyes (23). To reduce the risk of bleeding during the procedure, where applicable, patients should be advised to stop taking their warfarin at least 48 hours before the PCI (16). Then, on the day of the procedure, a blood sample should be checked to ensure that the international normalised ratio (INR) is less than 2, because if the patient's anticoagulation status is higher than that, it increases their risk of bleeding (5). Patients at increased risk of systemic thromboembolism on withdrawal of warfarin, such as those with mitral valve disease or a prior history of systemic thromboembolism, may be admitted to hospital for a few days prior to the procedure to be anticoagulated with heparin, while the warfarin is stopped (5). If the patient is on intravenous unfractionated heparin, it may be stopped 4 hours prior to the procedure (27). Alternatively, depending on the cardiologist's preference, this can be continued until the patient's arrival in the cath lab. The ACT can then be measured, which will help in calculating how much bolus of intravenous heparin will need to be administered for the procedure (17).

On the day of the procedure, the nurse should check that the above details have been completed, and then record baseline observations, such as blood pressure, pulse, temperature and blood glucose, if the patient is diabetic (5). A venflon should be inserted into their arm so that the necessary drugs can be administered during and after the procedure. The nurse should check that the patient has shaved appropriately. A patient identity band, a pair of modesty (paper) pants and a theatre gown will be provided and the patient will be asked to change into them for the procedure (30).

Patients should be fasted as per hospital protocol. Prior to any elective surgery, patients are usually fasted to reduce anaesthetic/sedation-induced pulmonary aspiration. In general, clear fluids are allowed up to 2 hours before anaesthesia and light meals up to 6 hours (22). The American Society of Anaesthesiologists recommends that patients undergoing local analgesia procedures such as cardiac catheterisation should have the same restrictions as those undergoing general anaesthesia. These guidelines are arbitrary and based upon a consensus opinion (22). As prolonged fasting increases patient discomfort, resulting in thirst, nausea, headache, hypoglycaemia, feeling faint and dizziness, the hospital protocol may not follow these guidelines. As the risk of a patient undergoing emergency CABG surgery as a result of PCI is less than 1%, many units in the United Kingdom do not fast their patients prior to the procedure (17; 22). As the contrast dye used in the procedure is nephrotoxic, patients with an increased risk, such as those with renal impairment or low cardiac output, should be started on intravenous fluids prior to the procedure if they are fasting (16).

In order to reduce anxiety, the nurse may inform the patient and their family about the procedure and what to expect, and answer any questions that they may have. However, it is the cardiologist responsible for the procedure who should obtain written consent from the patient after fully explaining the procedure, including its risks and benefits (5).

Anxiety may provoke angina before the start of the procedure, or the patient may drop their blood pressure and feel faint on arrival in the cath lab (23). Therefore, depending on the hospital protocol, the patient may receive a mild sedative prior to the procedure. The nurse should ensure that the written consent has been obtained prior to administering it (16). Oral diazepam of 5–20 mg can be given to adults orally 1–2 hours prior to the procedure or diazemuls may be given intravenously just prior to the procedure (23).

During the percutaneous coronary intervention

Once the patient arrives in the cath lab, they will be asked to lie down on the catheterisation table. Electrode stickers will be placed on their torso so that the ECG can monitor their heart rate and rhythm throughout the procedure (13). A probe may be placed on the patient's finger to monitor their blood oxygen saturations and their blood pressure will be monitored intravascularly throughout the procedure. Unless it is against the patient's religious beliefs, the staff will ensure that the proposed access area has been shaved properly (13).

Although access for the majority of PCIs is obtained via the femoral artery (known as the Judkin's approach), it can also be obtained via the brachial artery (known as the Sones procedure) or the radial artery (16). The cardiologist will decide prior to the procedure and inform the patient which artery will be used to gain access. Once the patient is lying on the table, the selected access artery will be liberally cleaned with an antiseptic solution. Then, the patient will be covered with sterile drapes, leaving the access artery uncovered. Once the preparations to make the patient sterile are completed, liberal amounts of local anaesthetic will be applied to the selected site (16). The patient should be warned that they may experience some burning as the anaesthetic is being injected (2).

Once the area is anaesthetised, an introducer sheath is inserted into the artery. The patient may feel some tugging and pushing around this time. Usually, there is a small spurt of blood out initially, which shows the physician that the sheath is in the artery (16). The introducer sheath has a one-way valve system, which allows the physician to insert the guide wires and balloon catheters. This minimises bleeding at the puncture site and reduces stabbing the artery every time a catheter needs to be inserted (16). Although most patients experience little or no discomfort during the procedure, patients should be advised to let staff know if the local anaesthetic begins to wear off so that more may be given (30). Patients should also be advised to let the staff know if they are experiencing any angina or chest pain so that suitable analgesia can be administered (30).

A guidewire is inserted through the introducer sheath and advanced to the aortic arch. The guiding catheter is then advanced along the guidewire to the appropriate coronary ostium (the opening of the coronary artery). Then, the guidewire is removed (16). The guiding catheter has a bifurcated adapter with two ports. One provides access for the insertion and removal of the PCI catheters. The other port is used for injecting the radio-opaque contrast dye into the coronary artery and measuring the aortic pressure (16). Unlike a ventriculogram, in which large amounts of contrast are injected to measure the ventricles, patients rarely get the tingles and hot-flush feeling associated with contrast dye during a PCI (23).

A baseline angiogram is usually performed first in order to evaluate any changes in the coronary arteries since the diagnostic angiogram, such as the development of a total occlusion or thrombus, and also to obtain more views of the coronary arteries to help in deciding which coronary intervention would be best, such as whether to just do a PTCA or whether a rotablation would be more appropriate (2).

After confirming that the lesion is still suitable for PCI, it is measured for appropriate balloon sizing. Then, the patient is anticoagulated with heparin or bivalirudin to prevent clots from forming on or in the catheter system during the procedure (16). Intracoronary nitrates may be administered to reduce the risk of coronary spasm throughout the procedure (2).

Although an angioplasty catheter has a balloon or a combination of balloon and stent on it, it is considerably smaller than the guiding catheter. A guidewire is initially inserted through the guiding catheter across the stenotic area. The angioplasty catheter is then inserted through the guiding catheter, along the guidewire to the area of the lesion. Radio-opaque markers at each end of the balloon are used to centre the balloon/stent in the appropriate position. Once the balloon/stent is placed correctly within the area to be treated, the balloon on the PCl catheter is inflated several times. A balloon may be inflated for 60–120 seconds, as tolerated; stents may be inflated for 10–20 seconds (13). Patients may feel chest pain at this time, similar to their angina. This may be eased by the deflation of the balloon or intravenous painkillers (23).

Complications such as vessel recoil and abrupt closure occur most often during this early phase; however, their incidence is low and re-dilation can be performed readily at this time. After dilation and stenting are complete, the balloon dilation catheter is removed. Another angiogram taken at 30° and 60° is completed and 'freeze frame' pictures are taken to define more clearly the results of the procedure. Then, the guiding catheter is removed (16).

Post percutaneous coronary intervention

Once the procedure is completed, the patient will be escorted back to the ward. On warding, the patient is attached to a cardiac monitor and blood pressure cuff so that the nurse can obtain their baseline observations. The nurse will check their puncture site, to observe any bleeding, check the pedal pulse and the peripheral skin colour and temperature of the limb below the puncture site (16). If the femoral artery is used, the nurse will check the pedal pulse on the affected leg or the radial pulse on the affected arm following a Brachial procedure. A 12-lead ECG should be completed to establish a baseline if the patient's condition should change suddenly (16).

Patients identified as having a high risk for restenosis or unstable lesions may be started on an intravenous GP IIa/IIIb antagonist (16). Therefore, patients may come back to the ward still attached to an intravenous pump. They may have to remain attached to the pump for up to 12 hours after the procedure, depending on which GP IIa/IIIb agent was prescribed.

The patient is allowed to eat and drink immediately after the procedure. Patients should be encouraged to drink plenty of fluid following the procedure in order to compensate for the diuretic action of the contrast dye, as well as to flush out the myocardial and vascular depressant drugs in their system, and to prevent hypotension. If the patient is unable to drink, intravenous fluids should be administered (2).

As anticoagulants are used during PCI, patients may be warded with the introducer sheath (known as a femoral sheath) still in their groin if the femoral artery was used for access. If bivalirudin is the anticoagulant used, the femoral sheath can be removed 2 hours after the bivalirudin has been discontinued (9). If heparin was used during the procedure, the femoral sheath should be removed as per hospital protocol, whether that is waiting until the ACT reaches a certain level or just waiting until 3–4 hours after the procedure (9; 17). The sheath may be removed using manual pressure or compression devices (see Chapter 2). Depending on hospital protocol, the patient must continue complete bed rest for 3–6 hours after the sheath(s) is removed (16; 25). During the time that the femoral sheath is in the femoral artery, the patient may have their head elevated by about 30°; however, they should be advised to keep the affected leg straight (9). Once the femoral sheath is removed, the patient should be advised to lie flat for the first 2 hours but can sit up for the remainder of the recommended bed rest.

Unfortunately, using a vascular closure device such as an AngioSeal has not reduced the risks associated with puncture-site complications. Therefore, even if the femoral sheath has been removed at the end of the procedure and a vascular device used to achieve haemostasis, patients should be closely monitored for several hours and nurses should continue to monitor the puncture site and pedal pulse as they would for patients without a vascular device (15; 17). Whilst the patient is on bed rest, the nurse should observe the access site every half-hour for signs of bleeding, swelling or haematoma formation (16). Patients should be advised to keep their leg straight and press over the puncture site before coughing or sneezing. They should inform nursing staff if they feel any blood, wetness or stickiness (13). As tachycardia and hypotension can indicate that the patient is losing blood, which may not be visible if it is a retroperitoneal bleed, the heart rate and blood pressure should be recorded half-hourly. Often, a patient complaining of low backache is the first symptom of a retroperitoneal bleed (16).

It is important to avoid hypotension post PCI and stenting, as a fall in systemic blood pressure reduces coronary perfusion pressure and a thrombus could form in the stent. Therefore, if a patient drops their systemic pressure below 90 mmHg, it should be corrected with intravenous saline or Gelofusine and the foot of the bed elevated. In addition, if the patient is bradycardic, intravenous atropine of 0.6–1.2 mg may be required (13; 23).

Patients should be asked to inform the nursing staff if they feel any chest pain post procedure, as it may indicate either the start of vasospasm or impending occlusion. Angina may be described as a burning, squeezing heaviness or as sharp, mid-sternal pain. Other signs and symptoms of myocardial ischaemia include ischaemic ECG changes (elevation of the ST segments or T-wave inversion), dysrhythmias, hypotension and nausea. The doctor should be informed of these problems, as it is difficult to distinguish between transient vasospasm and acute occlusion. If the chest pain is a transient vasospasm, it can be relieved by vasodilation therapy, such as administering glycerine trinitrate (GTN). However, this would be unsuitable for severely hypotensive patients (16).

Therefore, if a patient complains of angina post PCI, they should immediately be commenced on oxygen via a facemask or nasal cannula. A 12-lead ECG should be recorded to document any acute changes. If the angina resolves and any acute ECG changes caused by medical therapy disappear, it is safe to assume that a transient vasospasm episode occurred; however, if the angina continues and the ECG changes persist, particularly ST elevation, re-dilation or emergency CABG surgery should be considered (16).

Diabetic patients should be advised to omit their metformin for 48 hours post cardiac catheterisation procedures (6). As metformin should only be restarted after the renal function has been re-evaluated and found to be normal, the patient should ask their family doctor to check their urea and electrolytes (17).

If no complications occur, patients may be discharged the next day. Although, with less complex lesions, patients who have not received a GP IIa/IIIb antagonist may be discharged on the same day, depending on the cardiologist's discretion. Patients can usually resume their normal routine within several days (13).

DISCHARGE ADVICE

In order to protect the puncture site from bleeding, patients should be advised:

1. To feel the puncture site for signs of a growing lump over the next 2–3 days. If one develops or they get pins and needles in that leg, they should come back to their local hospital to have it scanned.
2. That they may get a bruise around the puncture site and normally this gets bigger as gravity pulls it down the leg. Unless it is painful, they should not worry about this.
3. That there may be a little bit of blood staining on their underwear. If the blood is bright red and spurting, they should send for an ambulance. Whilst waiting for the ambulance, they should lie down on a firm surface and press firmly just above the puncture site.

4. That it is very rare for problems like these to occur but, in order to minimise them, they should:
   - shower in preference to bathing for the next 2–3 days. If they only have a bath, they should use tepid water (30);
   - not scrub vigorously over the puncture site;
   - avoid heavy lifting and pulling for the next 2–3 days (30);
   - avoid driving for a week – the DVLA (2006) recommends no driving for a week after the procedure for group 1 drivers. People who drive large lorries and buses fall into group 2 and are not allowed to drive for a minimum of 6 weeks after a PCI. They will need to have an assessment and an exercise test before they can recommence commercial driving (8).

CARE PLANS

NURSING CONSIDERATION BEFORE THE PROCEDURE

The principle preparations for PCI are the same as those for any surgical procedure. The primary aim of nursing care is, therefore, to maximise patient safety and comfort during the procedure and to optimise conditions for a successful outcome. This is achieved by ensuring that the patient is physically and psychologically prepared for the procedure, and that all documentation, including laboratory results and reports, are available to the cath lab staff (7).

PRE-PROCEDURE CARE PLAN FOR PATIENTS UNDERGOING A PERCUTANEOUS CORONARY INTERVENTION

Action	Rationale
Obtain a brief history and check that biographical details and next of kin are correct	Checking the patient's biographical details and next of kin ensures that medical records are up-to-date and that, in the event of an emergency, the correct person is contacted. Record keeping is a fundamental part of nursing care, ensuring high standards of clinical care and improving communication and dissemination of information (18)
Explain to the patient and their family what a PCI is and what will happen during and after the procedure. Provide an information booklet about the procedure	The period before an invasive procedure may be a time of anxiety and fear, for various reasons. Discussion and reassurance may help to relieve some of these feelings (10)

Action	Rationale
Check whether the patient is allergic to any food, drugs or other substances. Inform the doctor if the patient is allergic to any potential drugs used in the procedure	Patients with a history of allergy to iodine-containing substances, such as seafood or contrast agents, should be given an antihistamine and steroids before the procedure (30). In addition to this, a non-ionic contrast dye may be used for the procedure (5)
Check the medication regime. Metformin should be stopped 24 hours before the procedure	Metformin-associated lactic acidosis can be precipitated by the contrast dye used during the procedure. Although, in patients without renal failure, metformin can be used up to the day of contrast administration, ideally, it should be avoided 24 hours prior to the procedure (6; 23)
Nephrotoxic drugs and non-steroidal anti-inflammatory drugs should be avoided for a few days prior to the procedure	High doses of contrast dye may cause contrast-induced nephropathy. In order to minimise renal complications, it is advisable to avoid nephrotoxic drugs and non-steroidal anti-inflammatory drugs for several days prior to the procedure (6)
Warfarin should be stopped at least 48 hours prior to the procedure	Warfarin should be withheld for at least 48 hours prior to the procedure, to ensure an INR of less than 2. Patients at high risk of thromboembolism should be admitted for heparinisation while the effects of oral anticoagulation wane (5)
Ideally, INR should be less than 2 (inform the cardiologist if it is higher)	Warfarin interferes with blood coagulation by blocking the effect of vitamin K. It has a long-acting half-life of 36–42 hours. The anticoagulation effect is described in a measurement of the INR. Therefore, any INR measurement of more than 2 increases the patient's risk of bleeding uncontrollably during and/or after the procedure (3)
If the patient is on low-molecular-weight heparin, the	The half-life of a low-molecular-weight heparin administered subcutaneously

Action	Rationale
last injection should be given at least 12 hours prior to the procedure	is about 4 hours (3). Therefore, if prescribed, the morning dose should be omitted prior to the procedure in order to reduce the risk of bleeding (17)
Check that a recent full blood count and urea and electrolyte blood results are available	Severe anaemia (Hb < 8) and/or severe electrolyte imbalance are contraindicators for PCI (5; 13). The cause of anaemia should be identified and treated prior to the procedure (13). Low potassium results in increased sensitivity and excitability of the myocardium, which may predispose to arrhythmias (13; 16). Elevation in serum creatinine may indicate problems with kidney function (16). As patients with renal failure have an increased risk of developing contrast nephropathy, risks versus benefits must be considered, and the patient should be hydrated during and after the procedure (2; 6)
Record ECG, blood pressure, pulse, temperature and blood glucose	This information should be evaluated to ensure that the patient is suitable for the procedure (5). It is also used to act as a baseline to compare the patient's vital signs with after the procedure (30)
Check for patent left and right pedal pulse	This information will be used for comparison in evaluating peripheral pulses after the catheterisation procedure (30)
Cannulate the patient	To provide intravenous access to administer prescribed drugs and fluids (13; 30)
If it is not against the patient's religious beliefs, ensure that the patient has shaved their groin appropriately	Body hair is removed in order to reduce infection risk during catheterisation (13; 30). Although most catheterisations are usually performed from the right femoral artery, it is expedient to routinely prepare both groins in case of difficulties in catheter advancement

Action	Rationale
	which may force a switch to the other groin once the procedure has begun (2)
Record the patient's height and weight	The amount of some of the drugs prescribed during the procedure may be calculated on the patient's body weight (2; 30)
The patient should be advised of the hospital's pre-procedure fasting protocol	Gastric emptying of water and non-caloric fluids has an average half-time of 10 minutes. Gastric emptying of solids depends on the caloric density of the meal; therefore, patients are usually advised to have a light meal before they start fasting (22)
Patients may wear dentures, glasses and hearing aids during the procedure	Patients are better able to communicate when dentures and hearing aids are in place. Glasses allow the patient to view the procedure better and help to keep the patient oriented to the surroundings (13; 30)
Allow patients to empty their bladder before the procedure	To help make them more comfortable (30)
Ensure that the informed consent has been signed prior to the procedure	This is a legal requirement (17)
If the patient is a female of child-bearing age, she may be asked by the radiographer to sign a form indicating her pregnancy status	Pregnancy is a relative contraindicator in cardiac catheterisation procedures (13). However, as direct irradiation of the uterus can usually be avoided in procedures that involve structures above the diaphragm, fluoroscopic procedures on pregnant women may be justifiable in an emergency situation (2)

POST-PROCEDURE CARE PLAN

Goal/aim of care

The nursing care of patients following PCI is directed towards the prevention and detection of complications (30).

Action	Rationale
On warding, attach the patient to a cardiac monitor and check pulse and blood pressure	In order to observe the patient's vital signs post procedure (16)
Monitoring the pulse	Tachycardia (100–120 beats per minute) is not unusual after catheterisation. This may be a sign of anxiety, an indication of fluid loss due to diuresis, or a reaction to medication used during the procedure, such as atropine. Fluids, time and reassurance often bring the heart rate down to more normal levels. Heart rates above 120 beats per minute should be evaluated for other causes, such as haemorrhage, more severe fluid imbalance, fever or arrhythmias (30). If not on betablockers, a bradycardia may indicate a vasovagal response, arrhythmias or an infarction and should be assessed by an ECG and correlated with other clinical signs, such as pain and blood pressure (30)
Blood pressure	Patients may return to the ward with a low blood pressure caused by drugs, such as vasodilators, administered during the procedure. In addition, the contrast dye acts as an osmotic diuretic and patients may become hypotensive due to volume depletion. Patients are thus kept on bed rest until fluid balance is restored, with oral liquids or by intravenous replacement. If the blood pressure is less than 75–80% of baseline, other causes such as blood loss or arrhythmias must be considered and assessed, and the doctor notified (30)
Pedal pulse	The most frequent complication of PCI is arterial thrombosis. The puncture site in the groin should be checked for visible bleeding, swelling or tenderness.

Action	Rationale
	The arterial pulse at the site and at points distal to it should be compared with pulses on the opposite limb and those recorded before the procedure. Capillary filling and the warmth of the limb should also be evaluated. Blanching, cramping, coolness, pain, numbness or tingling may indicate reduced perfusion and must be carefully evaluated. A diminished or absent pulse is a sign of serious arterial occlusion (13; 30). If a compression device is being used to achieve haemostasis, the pressure should be reduced. If this does not improve circulation, medical staff should be informed (30)
Check the puncture site for signs of bleeding or haematoma	Research shows that the majority of bleeding/haematoma was detected by nurses checking the groin (4)
Until the patient is mobile, check these observations half-hourly and ask the patient to report any feelings of wetness, stickiness, warmth or bleeding in the puncture-site area	Research shows that a large proportion of puncture-site bleeding was detected through the patient's calling for assistance (4)
Advise the patient to keep the affected leg straight whilst on bed rest	Bleeding and haematoma formation may occur when a patient moves the limb too vigorously (13; 30)
Ensure that a post-procedure ECG has been completed	The pre and post ECGs may be used for comparison if the patient develops any chest pain or arrhythmias (13; 16)
If the patient is a diabetic, check their blood sugar on warding	To ensure that the patient is not hypoglycaemic, as they may have fasted for long periods prior to the procedure (30)
Ensure any intravenous pumps are running at the correct rate, and administer any drugs prescribed post procedure	It is the ward nurses' responsibility to ensure that the prescribed drugs, intravenous or oral, are administered correctly (16; 19)

Action	Rationale
The patient can sit up at a 30° angle until the femoral sheaths are removed	Research has shown that no difference in bleeding at the catheter-insertion site was observed whether the patient was lying flat or if the bed head was elevated by 30° (9; 17)
Encourage the patient to drink and provide something to eat	Patients are often tired, hungry and uncomfortable when they return from the laboratory (30). Patients should be encouraged to drink plenty in order to prevent hypotension (2)
Observe urine output, as a poor urine output may be the first indication of contrast-induced renal failure	Contrast nephropathy is a recognised complication of procedures that use contrast dye (6) and a poor urine output is an early indication of this condition (13). However, as the contrast dye acts as an osmotic diuretic, patients may have an increase in urine output for a short time after the procedure (30)
If a vascular closure device was used to achieve haemostasis, such as an AngioSeal, please follow the manufacturer's guidelines about bed rest and mobilising the patient	Although these devices have been shown to reduce the time taken to obtain haemostasis (2; 13), the patient maintains the risk of developing cardiac complications such as bradycardia or hypotension as a result of the drugs used during the procedure (30); therefore, it is good policy to maintain cardiac monitoring for at least 4 hours after the PCI (15)
Whilst on bed rest, advise patients to press on the puncture site if they cough or sneeze, and to inform the nurse if they experience any chest pain	Patients are advised to press on the puncture site while coughing or sneezing in order to prevent the newly formed clot from being disturbed (4). Chest pain may indicate potential cardiac complications; therefore, nurses should be aware of it if it is present (16)
If the patient has the femoral sheaths in situ, the cardiologists will advise when the sheaths should be removed	Femoral sheaths are normally removed 3–4 hours after catheterisation procedures that utilised heparin, to allow time for the heparin to dissipate (16; 17)

Action	Rationale
After the femoral sheath has been removed from the femoral artery and haemostasis has been achieved, the patient should remain on bed rest as per hospital protocol	Patients are advised to remain on bed rest in order not to disturb the newly formed clot (12). Bed-rest post-sheath removal guidelines vary from hospital to hospital (25). Keeling *et al.* (2000) suggest that lying the patient flat for 2 hours and then sitting them up for 2 hours is usually sufficient to ensure haemostasis (12). However, smaller studies since then indicate that it may be safe to reduce bed rest further (25)
Once mobile, observations may cease, unless the patient complains of numbness, pins and needles or a lump in the groin area, or the puncture site begins to bleed	Complications such as bleeding or haematomas are normally observed within 10 minutes of ambulation (14)
Advise patients to take things slowly when they first mobilise	A patient may drop their blood pressure by simply standing up abruptly after prolonged bed rest (28)
Prior to discharge, the patient should be instructed about puncture-site care, and informed of any signs and symptoms which require a doctor's review. A discharge leaflet should be provided	So that patients will be aware of potential complications post discharge and know what to do in the event of these occurring (13)
Any changes in medication should be discussed with the patient	When discharging a patient, it is the nurses' responsibility to inform the patient about the medication that they have been prescribed so that they will take it correctly at home (19)
If the patient normally takes metformin, they should be advised to have their urea and electrolytes checked by their family doctor 48 hours after the procedure and restart it when advised to do so by them	Metformin is contraindicated in patients with renal dysfunction, as determined by elevated serum creatinine levels. Therefore, metformin should only be resumed after the renal function is found to be normal (17)

REFERENCES

1. Al-Obaidi, M., Noble, M. and Siva, A. (2004) *Crash Course Cardiology*, 2nd edn, London, Mosby.
2. Baim, D. S. (2006) *Grossman's Cardiac Catheterisation: Angiography and Intervention*, 7th edn, Philadelphia, PA, Lippincott Williams & Wilkins.
3. Blann, A., Landray, M. and Lip, G. (2002) 'An overview of antithrombotic therapy', *British Medical Journal*, **325**: 762–5.
4. Botti, M., Williamson, B. and Steen, K. (2001) 'Coronary angiography observations: Evidence-based or ritualistic practice?', *Heart & Lung: The Journal of Acute and Critical Care*, **30**(2): 138–45.
5. Braunweld, E., Zipes, D. and Libby, P. (2001) *Heart Disease: A Textbook of Cardiovascular Medicine*, Vol. 1, 6th edn, London, W.B. Saunders Co.
6. Brinker, J. A., Davidson, C. J. and Laskey, W. (2005) 'Preventing in-hospital cardiac and renal complications in high-risk PCI patients', *European Heart Journal Supplements*, **7** (Suppl G): G13–25, available online at *www.eurheartj/sui054*.
7. Carter, L. and Lamerton, M. (1996) 'Understanding balloon mitral valvuloplasty: The Inoue technique', *Intensive and Critical Care Nursing*, **12**: 147–54.
8. DVLA (2006) *For Medical Practitioners: At a Glance Guide to the Current Medical Standards of Fitness to Drive*, February, available online at *www.dvla.gov.uk*.
9. Galli, G. (2005) 'Ask the experts: Re removing arterial and venous sheaths after PCI', *Critical Care Nurse*, available online at *www.findarticles.com*.
10. Hughes, S. (2002) 'The effects of pre-operative information', *Nursing Standard*, **16**: 28, 33–7.
11. Julian, D. G., Cowan, J. C. and McLenachan, J. M. (2005) *Cardiology*, 8th edn, London, Elsevier Saunders.
12. Keeling, A., Fisher, C., Haugh, K., Powers, E. and Turner, M. (2000) 'Reducing time in bed after percutaneous transluminal coronary angioplasty (TIBS III)', *American Journal of Critical Care*, **9**(3): 185–7.
13. Kern, M. (2003) *The Cardiac Catheterisation Handbook*, 4th edn, London, Mosby.
14. Logemann, T., Luetmer, P., Kaliebe, J., Olson, K. and Murdock, D. (1999) 'Two versus six hours of bed rest following left-sided cardiac catheterisation and a meta-analysis of early ambulation trials', *The American Journal of Cardiology*, **84**: 486–8.
15. Montalsecot, G., Andersen, H., Antoniucer, D., Betriu, A., de Boer, M., Grip, L., *et al.* (2004) 'Recommendations on percutaneous coronary intervention for the reperfusion of acute ST elevation myocardial infarction', *Heart*, 90, available online at *http://heart.bmjjournals.com/cgi/content/full/90/6/e37*.
16. Morton, P. G., Fontaine, D. K., Hudak, C. M. and Gallo, B. M. (2005) *Critical Care Nursing: A Holistic Approach*, 8th edn, Philadelphia, PA, Lippincott Williams & Wilkins.
17. Norell, M. and Perrins, J. (2003) *Essential Interventional Cardiology*, Philadelphia, PA, W.B. Saunders Co.
18. Nursing Midwifery Council (2002a) *Guidelines for Records and Record Keeping*, London, Nursing and Midwifery Council, April.
19. Nursing Midwifery Council (2002b) *Guidelines for the Administration of Medicines*, London, Nursing and Midwifery Council.
20. Popma, J. J., Berger, P., Ohman, E. M., Harrington, R. A., Grines, C. and Weitz, J. I. (2004) 'The Seventh ACCP Conference on Antithrombotic and Thrombolytic Therapy', *Chest*, **126**(3 Suppl): 575S–99S.
21. Sennik, D. (2005) 'POEM review: Aspirin and PPI is safer than clopidogrel if patient has history of GI bleeding', available online at *www.druginfozone.nhs.uk*.
22. Soreide, E., Eriksson, L. I., Hirlekar, G., Eriksson, H., Henneberg, W., Sandin, R., Raeder (Task Force on Scandinavian Pre-operative Fasting Guidelines, Clinical

Practice Committee Scandinavian Society of Anaesthesiology and Intensive Care Medicine) (2005) 'Pre-operative fasting guidelines: An update', *Acta Anaesthesiologica Scandinavica*, **49**: 1041–7.

23. Swanton, R. H. (2003) *Pocket Consultant Cardiology*, 5th edn, Oxford, Blackwell Publishing.
24. Swee Choon, N. G. (2006) 'Understanding balloon angioplasty', *The Star Online*.
25. Tagney, J. and Lackie, D. (2005) 'Bed-rest post-femoral arterial sheath removal: What is safe practice? A clinical audit', *Nursing in Critical Care*, **10**(4): 167–73.
26. Tcheng, J. and Kindsvater, D. (2005) 'Hospital percutaneous coronary intervention volume and outcome: Does it matter?', *Journal in Interventional Cardiology*, **18**(1): 17–19.
27. Thompson, P. (1997) *Coronary Care Manual*, London, Churchill Livingstone.
28. Topol, E. J. (1999) *Textbook of Interventional Cardiology*, 3rd edn, London, W.B. Saunders Co.
29. Tortora, G. J. and Derrickson, B. (2006) *Principles of Anatomy and Physiology*, 8th edn, Chichester, John Wiley and Sons Inc.
30. Woods, S., Froelicher, E. and Motzer, S. (2000) *Cardiac Nursing*, 4th edn, Philadelphia, PA, Lippincott Williams & Wilkins.

6 Percutaneous Balloon Mitral Valvuloplasty

MITRAL VALVE

The mitral valve is an atrioventricular valve, which sits between the left atrium and the left ventricle. It is bicuspid, indicating that it has two leaflets (18). When the ventricles are relaxed, the ventricular pressure is low and the pointed ends of the cusps project into the ventricle opening, allowing blood flow from the left atrium to the left ventricle (27). When the ventricles contract, the pressure of the blood drives the cusps upward until their edges meet and close the opening, thus preventing blood back-flowing into the left atrium. At the same time, the papillary muscles, which are attached to the mitral valve leaflets by tendon-like fibrous cords called chordae tendinae (see Figure 6.1), are also contracting, thus pulling on and tightening the chordae tendinae. This prevents the valve cusps from everting or swinging upward into the atria, which ensures that blood flows through the heart in one direction only (27).

MITRAL STENOSIS

Mitral stenosis is a serious cardiac condition. It occurs as a long-term consequence of rheumatic fever, whereby, as a result of inflammation, the valve cusps become thickened and fibrous; it is characterised by the fusion of one or both commissures. The valve leaflets may be thickened, fibrous and calcified, causing reduced mobility, and the chordae tendinae may also thicken and shorten. This results in a small, oval, central valve orifice, which impedes the blood flow from the left atrium to the left ventricle (7). As the left atrial pressure rises, the left atrium enlarges and pulmonary congestion occurs. As a result of the enlarged atrium, atrial fibrillation may develop and the left ventricular filling becomes more dependent on the left atrial contraction. These abnormalities usually become haemodynamically significant when the patient enters their 40s and 50s (18; 21).

The primary aim of treatment in mitral stenosis is to reduce left atrial pressure in order to reduce pulmonary congestion and thereby improve dyspnoea. Invariably, initial therapy is medical (7). Severe mitral stenosis has traditionally been treated with surgical splitting or replacement of the mitral valve (7). However,

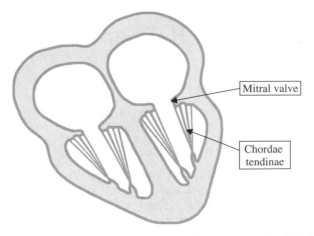

Figure 6.1. The mitral valve and chordae tendinae on the left side.

percutaneous techniques as alternatives to surgery for the treatment of valvular disease were introduced in the early 1980s (16). Patients with pure mitral stenosis without mitral regurgitation or mitral valve calcification are considered suitable for treatment with percutaneous balloon mitral valvuloplasty (PBMV). It can be performed in any age group but the results are better in the younger age group, in whom the chordae tendinae have not shortened and thickened. A PBMV can be performed when necessary during the mid-trimester of pregnancy (24).

Although several techniques have been developed to perform a PBMV, the Inoue balloon catheter technique has become the procedure of choice for treating mitral stenosis (8) as it has been proven to provide easy access and is reliable. Clinical success is high and complication rates are low (16). During the procedure, a balloon is passed from the right femoral vein into the right atrium, through the atrial septum into the left atrium using the trans-septal technique. Using fluoroscopy and radio-opaque markers, the balloon is positioned across the mitral valve. As the balloon is inflated, it causes controlled tearing of the adhesions that are holding the valve leaflets together at the commissures, which partially relieves the obstruction (13) (see Figure 6.2).

POTENTIAL COMPLICATIONS

Overall, PBMV is a low-risk procedure when performed by experienced operators on properly selected patients, with a reported mortality of 0.5%. The main causes of death are left ventricular perforation or the poor initial condition of the patient (21). The trans-septal puncture may result in a cardiac tamponade (2%) or atrial septal defect. Although an atrial septal defect with left-to-right shunting was detectable in 8–87% of patients, this depended on the sensitivity of the

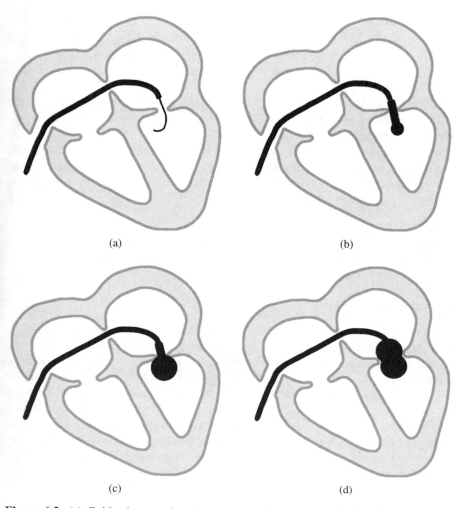

(a) (b)

(c) (d)

Figure 6.2. (a) Guidewire crossing the trans-septal puncture and going into the mitral valve. (b) The balloon is passed through the mitral valve into the left ventricle. (c) The balloon is partially inflated and is pulled back into the mitral orifice. (d) The balloon is inflated, stretching the stenotic mitral valve.

methods used for detection and the majority were clinically unimportant, as they decreased or disappeared during follow-up (16).

An embolic stroke may occur in 1–2% of patients (16). It may be caused by the displacement of thrombus from the left atrium. This risk can be minimised by anticoagulation for several weeks prior to the procedure and scanning the left atrium using a transoesophageal echocardiogram before the PBMV (21).

Mild mitral regurgitation is fairly common (21). Severe mitral regurgitation ranges from 2 to 9%, and is usually caused by a tear in a valve cusp or in the chordae tendinae. Usually in these cases, one or both of the mitral commissures were too tightly fused to be split successfully by the balloon. Same-day surgical mitral valve replacement is necessary in about 2–3% of cases. Usually, even severe mitral valve regurgitation is well tolerated for a time by the patient, so elective surgery can be planned (1).

As PBMV catheters are larger, a 10–14 French introducer sheath may be used at the arterial or venous puncture sites. This increases the risk of bleeding or haematoma formation (20).

In addition to this, patients are at risk of other complications associated with percutaneous cardiac interventions, including arrhythmias, vascular damage, reaction to the contrast dye, congestive heart failure, infection, protamine reaction, vasovagal reaction and thrombosis (16; 21).

WHAT A PATIENT CAN EXPECT TO HAPPEN WHEN UNDERGOING A PERCUTANEOUS BALLOON MITRAL VALVULOPLASTY

PRIOR TO THE PBMV

In order to assess whether somebody is suitable for a PBMV, they will have to undergo some investigations. The preliminary, non-invasive investigations, such as physical examination, electrocardiogram (ECG), chest x-ray, transthoracic echocardiography and transoesophageal echocardiography, are normally carried out in the out-patients clinic, at the time of the pre-admission visit (7). The presence of broad notched P waves on an ECG recording reflects atrial hypertrophy associated with mitral valve stenosis. A chest x-ray can reveal the presence of calcium in or around the valve, left-ventricular or atrial hypertrophy, and pulmonary venous congestion and complete heart failure. A two-dimensional echocardiogram is used to scan the cardiac valves and chambers. A Doppler ultrasound study allows measurement of the transvalvular gradient, indirect calculation of the valve area and assessment of valvular regurgitation. With this information, the cardiologist is able to estimate the size of the valve orifice, visualise the degree of valve leaflet movement and determine the extent of left-ventricular or atrial hypertrophy (20).

As this is a percutaneous catheter procedure, the patient should be prepared for the procedure in a similar manner as that for a percutaneous coronary intervention (Chapter 5). However, prior to the PBMV, the patient must undergo a transoesophageal echocardiogram to assess the mitral valve structure and to exclude left atrial thrombus (16). Significant mitral regurgitation and thrombus in the left atrium, which might be dislodged during the trans-septal puncture, are absolute contraindications to PBMV (13). In practice, this is often performed during the 24 hours prior to the procedure. If it has not been performed, the patient should be fasted for 4–6 hours before the PBMV, as it may be performed during the procedure (21).

As atrial fibrillation is very common with mitral stenosis (3), the majority of patients will be anticoagulated with warfarin. Patients are normally advised to stop taking their warfarin 48 hours before the procedure. Then, on the day of the procedure, a blood sample should be checked to ensure that the international normalised ratio (INR) is less than 2, because if the patient's anticoagulation status is higher than that, it increases their risk of bleeding (5). Patients at increased risk of systemic thromboembolism on withdrawal from warfarin may be admitted to hospital for a few days prior to the procedure to be anticoagulated with heparin, while the warfarin is stopped (5). If the patient is on intravenous unfractionated heparin, it may be stopped 4 hours prior to the procedure (25). Alternatively, depending on the cardiologist's preference, this can be continued until the patient's arrival in the catheterisation laboratory (cath lab). The activated clotting time (ACT) can then be measured, which will help in calculating how much bolus of intravenous heparin will need to be administered for the procedure (21).

DURING THE PROCEDURE

PBMV is performed in the cardiac cath lab and involves many of the same steps as percutaneous coronary intervention (PCI) (see Chapter 5) (20). However, the percutaneous access site is usually the right groin, as the right femoral vein provides a direct approach from the inferior vena cava to the interatrial septum at the fossa ovalis. The fossa ovalis is where the original hole in the atrial septum, which people are born with, is, so it is easier to puncture this to cross the guidewire and valvuloplasty balloon into the left atrium (9).

The patient remains awake during the PBMV, although a mild sedative such as diazepam may be administered if the patient requires one (21). Once the right groin is anaesthetised, an introducer sheath is inserted into the right femoral artery to repeat the right and left heart catheterisation in order to determine the severity of any mitral regurgitation that may be present, and to assess the coronary arteries. For the patient, this has the advantage of combining invasive diagnostic investigations and treatment in one procedure. Occasionally, however, a patient will be prepared for PBMV, only to find that the invasive investigations reveal that they are not suitable for the procedure (7). The most likely reasons to preclude valvuloplasty are concomitant coronary artery disease requiring surgery or severe mitral regurgitation (7). Patients should be informed that the radio-opaque dye used during this part of the procedure may cause hot flushes, but they will only last a few seconds and are not painful (16).

Then, a large introducer sheath is inserted into the femoral vein. A trans-septal needle is guided through this via the vena cava into the right atrium. A trans-septal puncture is made close to, or in, the foramen ovale, so that the balloon catheter can cross the atrial septum and be guided into the mitral valve. Then, the balloon is inflated, stretching the valve. The patient may feel a little dizzy while the balloon is inflated, but this quickly resolves once the balloon is deflated (7). When the needle punctures the foramen ovale, there is a small risk (0.5–7%) that the atrium could be perforated, causing a tamponade, which is one of the reasons why it is important that the patient's INR is less than 2 prior to the procedure (21).

POST PROCEDURE

Post-procedure care is similar to the routine for percutaneous coronary intervention (PCI). The patient will be attached to a cardiac monitor, and the nurses will check the puncture site, pedal pulses and blood pressure half-hourly while the patient is on bed rest, to observe for any complications. In addition to observing for arrhythmias, vascular complications, systemic emboli and bleeding, the nurse should also observe for any signs of cardiac tamponade or mitral regurgitation (21). Both these complications require an urgent transthoracic echocardiogram to aid diagnosis (24).

If the patient has not been anaesthetised for a transoesophageal echocardiogram during the procedure, they are allowed to eat and drink immediately post procedure. Patients should be encouraged to drink plenty of fluid following the procedure in order to compensate for the diuretic action of the contrast dye, as well as to flush out the myocardial and vascular depressant drugs in their system, and to prevent hypotension. If the patient is unable to drink, intravenous fluids should be administered (1).

The patient can be discharged the day after the procedure unless there have been complications or they continue to require anticoagulation, usually for atrial fibrillation. Then, they may need to remain on heparin until their INR is at a therapeutic level, namely more than 2. This may be 48–72 hours post procedure (26). Normally, the introducer sheaths are removed 3–4 hours after a percutaneous procedure that uses heparin, so the effects of the heparin used during the procedure have waned in order to avoid prolonged compression (21). However, patients with a high risk of thromboembolism may have a continuous infusion of heparin following a PBMV. For these patients, the cardiologist will provide guidelines of when the sheaths should be removed. In view of the higher anticoagulation status of the patient, the person removing the sheath may prefer to use a compression device to manual pressure (21).

Depending on hospital protocol, the patient must continue complete bed rest for 4–6 hours after the sheath(s) is removed (20). During the time for which the introducer sheath is in the femoral artery, the patient may have their head elevated by about 30°; however, they should be advised to keep the affected leg straight (11). Once the femoral sheath is removed, the patient should be advised to lie flat for the first 2 hours but can sit up for the remainder of the recommended bed rest.

A further transthoracic echocardiogram may be performed before discharge, to exclude significant mitral regurgitation or residual left-to-right shunt and to provide a baseline assessment of residual stenosis, which assists future follow-up (21).

DISCHARGE ADVICE

In order to protect the puncture site from bleeding, patients should be advised:

1. To feel the puncture site for signs of a growing lump over the next 2–3 days. If one develops or they get pins and needles in that leg, they should come back to their local hospital to have it scanned.
2. That they may get a bruise around the puncture site and normally this gets bigger as gravity pulls it down the leg. Unless it is painful, they should not worry about this.
3. That there may be a little bit of blood staining on their underwear. If the blood is bright red and spurting, they should send for an ambulance. Whilst waiting for the ambulance, they should lie down on a firm surface and press firmly just above the puncture site.
4. That it is very rare for problems like these to occur but, in order to minimise them, patients should:

   - shower in preference to bathing for the next 2–3 days; if they only have a bath, they should use tepid water (28);
   - not scrub vigorously over the puncture site;
   - avoid heavy lifting and pulling for the next 2–3 days (28);
   - avoid driving for a week – the DVLA (2006) recommends no driving for a week after the procedure (10). If they hold a professional licence, they should advise the DVLA that they have had a PBMV, otherwise they do not need to inform them.

CARE PLANS

NURSING CONSIDERATION BEFORE THE PROCEDURE

The principle preparations for PBMV are the same as those for any surgical procedure. The primary aim of nursing care is, therefore, to maximise patient safety and comfort during the procedure and optimise conditions for a successful outcome. This is achieved by ensuring that the patient is physically and psychologically prepared for the procedure, and that all documentation, including laboratory results and reports, are available to the cath lab staff (7).

PRE-PROCEDURE CARE PLAN FOR PATIENTS UNDERGOING A
PERCUTANEOUS BALLOON MITRAL VALVULOPLASTY

Action	Rationale
Explain to the patient and their family what a mitral valvuloplasty is and what will happen during and after the procedure. Provide an information booklet about the procedure	The period before an invasive procedure may be a time of anxiety and fear, for various reasons. Discussion and reassurance may help to relieve some of these feelings (12)
Check whether the patient is allergic to any food, drugs or other substances. Inform the doctor if the patient is allergic to any potential drugs used in the procedure	Patients with a history of allergy to iodine-containing substances, such as seafood or contrast agents, should be given an antihistamine and steroids before the procedure (28). In addition to this, a non-ionic contrast dye may be used for the procedure (5)
Check the medication regime. Metformin should be stopped 24 hours before the procedure	Metformin-associated lactic acidosis can be precipitated by the contrast dye used during the procedure. Although, in patients without renal failure, metformin can be used up to the day of contrast administration, ideally, it should be avoided 24 hours prior to the procedure (6; 24)
Nephrotoxic drugs and non-steroidal anti-inflammatory drugs should be avoided for a few days prior to the procedure	High doses of contrast dye may cause contrast-induced nephropathy. In order to minimise renal complications, it is advisable to avoid nephrotoxic drugs and non-steroidal anti-inflammatory drugs for several days prior to the procedure (6)
Warfarin should be stopped at least 48 hours prior to the procedure	Warfarin should be withheld for at least 48 hours prior to the procedure, to ensure an INR of less than 2. Patients at high risk of thromboembolism should be admitted for heparinisation while the effects of oral anticoagulation wane (5)

Action	Rationale
Ideally, INR should be less than 2 (inform the cardiologist if it is higher)	Warfarin interferes with blood coagulation by blocking the effect of vitamin K. It has a long-acting half-life of 36–42 hours. The anticoagulation effect is described in a measurement of the INR. Therefore, any INR measurement more than 2 increases the patient's risk of bleeding uncontrollably during and/or after the procedure (2)
If the patient is on low-molecular-weight heparin, the last injection should be given at least 12 hours prior to the procedure	The half-life of a low-molecular-weight heparin administered subcutaneously is about 4 hours (2). Therefore, if prescribed, the morning dose should be omitted prior to the procedure in order to reduce the risk of bleeding (21)
Check that a recent full blood count, and urea and electrolyte blood results are available	Severe anaemia (Hb < 8) and/or severe electrolyte imbalance are contraindicators for PBMV (5; 16). The cause of anaemia should be identified and treated prior to the procedure (16). Low potassium results in increased sensitivity and excitability of the myocardium, which may predispose to arrhythmias (16; 20). Elevation in serum creatinine may indicate problems with kidney function (20). As patients with renal failure have an increased risk of developing contrast nephropathy, risks versus benefits must be considered, and the patient should be hydrated during and after the procedure (1; 6)
Record ECG, blood pressure, pulse, temperature and blood glucose	This information should be evaluated to ensure that the patient is suitable for the procedure (5). It is also used to act as a baseline to compare the patient's vital signs with after the procedure (28)

Action	Rationale
Check for patent left and right pedal pulse	This information will be used for comparison in evaluating peripheral pulses after the catheterisation procedure (28)
Cannulate the patient	To provide intravenous access to administer prescribed drugs and fluids (16; 28)
If it is not against the patient's religious beliefs, ensure that the patient has shaved their groin appropriately	Body hair is removed in order to reduce infection risk during catheterisation (16; 28). Although most catheterisations are usually performed from the right femoral artery, it is expedient to routinely prepare both groins in case of difficulties in catheter advancement which may force a switch to the other groin once the procedure has begun (1)
Record the patient's height and weight	The amount of some of the drugs prescribed during the procedure may be calculated on the patient's body weight (1; 28)
The patient should fast for at least 4–6 hours prior to the PBMV	The patient may need to have a transoesophageal echocardiogram prior to or during the PBMV (21)
Patients may wear dentures, glasses and hearing aids during the procedure	Patients are better able to communicate when dentures and hearing aids are in place. Glasses allow the patient to view the procedure better and help to keep the patient oriented to the surroundings (16; 28). These items can be removed by the lab staff if they decide to anaesthetise the patient for a transoesophageal echocardiogram
Ensure that identification and allergy bands are correct, legible and secure	To ensure correct identification and prevent possible problems (28)
Allow patients to empty their bladder before the procedure	To help make them more comfortable (28)

Action	Rationale
Ensure that consent is obtained by the doctor performing the procedure	Consent for any procedure must be obtained by the doctor performing the procedure and a patient signature obtained. A full explanation of the procedure should be given, outlining the benefits and risks (21)
If the patient is a female of child-bearing age, she may be asked by the radiographer to sign a form indicating her pregnancy status	Radiation from x-ray is contraindicated in pregnancy, especially in the first trimester, as it increases the risk of fetal central nerve damage, growth retardation, malformation or miscarriage. However, as direct irradiation of the uterus can usually be avoided in procedures that involve structures above the diaphragm, a PBMV can be performed when necessary during the mid-trimester of pregnancy. Extra precautions will be taken during fluoroscopy (1; 24)

POST-PROCEDURE CARE PLAN

Goal/aim of care

The nursing care of patients following PBMV is directed towards the prevention and detection of complications.

Action	Rationale
On warding, attach the patient to a cardiac monitor and check pulse and blood pressure	In order to observe the patient's vital signs post procedure (20)
Monitoring the pulse	Tachycardia (100–120 beats per minute) is not unusual after catheterisation. This may be a sign of anxiety, an indication of fluid loss due to diuresis or a reaction to medication used during the procedure, such as atropine. Fluids, time and reassurance often bring the

Action	Rationale
	heart rate down to more normal levels. Heart rates above 120 beats per min should be evaluated for other causes, such as haemorrhage, more severe fluid imbalance, fever or arrhythmias (28). If not on betablockers, a bradycardia may indicate a vasovagal response, arrhythmias or an infarction and should be assessed by an ECG and correlated with other clinical signs, such as pain and blood pressure (28)
Blood pressure	Patients may return to the ward with a low blood pressure caused by drugs, such as vasodilators, administered during the procedure. In addition, the contrast dye acts as an osmotic diuretic and patients may become hypotensive due to volume depletion. Patients are thus kept on bed rest until fluid balance is restored, with oral liquids or by intravenous replacement. If the blood pressure is less than 75–80% of baseline, other causes such as blood loss or arrhythmias must be considered and assessed, and the doctor notified (28)
If the patient has been anaesthetised, monitor the pulse oximetry	Hypoxia occurs for a variety of reasons following anaesthesia. The administration of supplemental oxygen in the immediate post-operative phase will help to reduce the risk of hypoxia occurring. The aim is to maintain normal levels of arterial blood gases and peripheral oxygen saturations (23)
If the patient has been anaesthetised, monitor the respiratory rate	Anaesthesia and opiates may depress respiration. Although the anaesthetist aims to have reversed these effects by the time the patient is warded,

Action	Rationale
	there is potential for severe respiratory depression to be present in the immediate post-procedure period (23)
Pedal pulse	The most frequent complication of a percutaneous procedure is arterial thrombosis. The puncture site in the groin should be checked for visible bleeding, swelling or tenderness. The arterial pulse at the site and at points distal to it should be compared with pulses on the opposite limb and those recorded before the procedure. Capillary filling and the warmth of the limb should also be evaluated. Blanching, cramping, coolness, pain, numbness or tingling may indicate reduced perfusion and must be carefully evaluated. A diminished or absent pulse is a sign of serious arterial occlusion (16; 28). If a compression device is being used to achieve haemostasis, the pressure should be reduced. If this does not improve circulation, medical staff should be informed (28)
Check the puncture site for signs of bleeding or haematoma	Research shows that the majority of bleeding/haematoma was detected by nurses checking the groin (4)
Until the patient is mobile, check these observations half-hourly and ask the patient to report any feelings of wetness, stickiness, warmth or bleeding in the puncture-site area	Research shows that a large proportion of puncture-site bleeding was detected through the patient's calling for assistance (4)
Advise the patient to keep the affected leg straight whilst on bed rest	Bleeding and haematoma formation may occur when a patient moves the limb too vigorously (16; 28)
Ensure that a post-procedure ECG has been completed	The pre and post ECGs may be used for comparison if the patient develops any chest pain or arrhythmias (16; 20)

Action	Rationale
If the patient is a diabetic, check their blood sugar on warding	To ensure that the patient is not hypoglycaemic, as they may have fasted for long periods prior to the procedure (28)
Ensure that any intravenous pumps are running at the correct rate, and administer any drugs prescribed post procedure	It is the ward nurses' responsibility to ensure that the prescribed drugs, intravenous or oral, are administered correctly (20; 22)
The patient can sit up at a 30° angle until the femoral sheaths are removed	Research has shown that no difference in bleeding at the catheter insertion site was observed whether the patient was lying flat or if the bed head was elevated by 30° (14; 21)
If the patient was anaesthetised, ensure that the patient is fully awake before providing them with something to eat or drink	During anaesthesia, voluntary muscular control is temporarily lost; therefore, post procedure, if the patient is not fully awake, fluids may be inhaled accidentally (23). Initially, try patients with sips of water
Once awake, encourage the patient to drink and provide them with something to eat	Patients are often tired, hungry and uncomfortable when they return from the laboratory (28). Patients should be encouraged to drink plenty in order to prevent hypotension (1)
Observe urine output, as a poor urine output may be the first indication of contrast-induced renal failure	Contrast nephropathy is a recognised complication of procedures that use contrast dye (6) and a poor urine output is an early indication of this condition (16). However, as the contrast dye acts as an osmotic diuretic, patients may have an increase in urine output for a short time after the procedure (28)
Advise patients to inform the nurse if they experience any chest pain	Chest pain may indicate potential cardiac complications; therefore, nurses should be aware of it if it is present (20)

Action	Rationale
If a vascular closure device was used to achieve haemostasis, such as an AngioSeal, please follow the manufacturer's guidelines about bed rest and mobilising the patient	Although these devices have been shown to reduce the time taken to obtain haemostasis (1; 16), the patient maintains the risk of developing cardiac complications such as bradycardia or hypotension as a result of the drugs used during the procedure (28); therefore, it is good policy to maintain cardiac monitoring for at least 4 hours after the procedure (19)
If the patient has the introducer sheath still in the femoral artery, cardiologists will advise when the sheaths should be removed	Although femoral sheaths are normally removed 3–4 hours after catheterisation procedures that utilise heparin (18), due to the high thrombo-embolic risk, femoral sheaths after a PBMV are taken out earlier and heparin continued for at least 24 hours, depending on the cardiologist's preference
Once the femoral sheath has been removed and haemostasis has been achieved, the patient must lie flat for 2 hours and then may sit up for 2 hours	Patients are advised to remain on bed rest in order not to disturb the newly formed clot over the puncture site. Research indicates that 4 hours' bed rest is sufficient to maintain the haemostasis (15)
Once mobile, observations may cease, unless the patient complains of numbness, pins and needles or a lump in the groin area or the puncture site begins to bleed	Complications such as bleeding or haematomas are normally observed within 10 minutes of ambulation (17)
Whilst on bed rest, advise the patient to press on the puncture site if they cough or sneeze	Patients are advised to press on the puncture site while coughing or sneezing in order to prevent the newly formed clot from being disturbed (4)
Advise patients to take things slowly when they first mobilise	A patient may drop their blood pressure by simply standing up abruptly after prolonged bed rest (26)

Action	Rationale
Prior to discharge, the patient should be instructed about puncture-site care, and informed of any signs and symptoms which require a doctor's review. A discharge leaflet should be provided	So that patients will be aware of potential complications post discharge and know what to do in the event of these occurring (16)
Any changes in medication should be discussed with the patient	When discharging a patient, it is the nurses' responsibility to inform the patient about the medication that they have been prescribed so that they will take it correctly at home (22)
If the patient normally takes metformin, they should be advised to have their urea and electrolytes checked by their family doctor 48 hours after the procedure and restart it when advised to by them	Metformin is contraindicated with patients with renal dysfunction, as determined by elevated serum creatinine levels. Therefore, metformin should only be resumed after the renal function is found to be normal (16)

REFERENCES

1. Baim, D. S. (2006) *Grossman's Cardiac Catheterisation: Angiography and Intervention*, 7th edn, Philadelphia, PA, Lippincott Williams & Wilkins.
2. Blann, A., Landray, M. and Lip, G. (2002) 'An overview of antithrombotic therapy', *British Medical Journal*, **325**: 762–5.
3. Boon, N. A. and Bloomfield, P. (2002) 'The medical management of valvar heart disease', *Heart*, **87**: 395–400.
4. Botti, M., Williamson, B. and Steen, K. (2001) 'Coronary angiography observations: Evidence-based or ritualistic practice?', *Heart & Lung: The Journal of Acute and Critical Care*, **30**(2): 138–45.
5. Braunweld, E., Zipes, D. and Libby, P. (2001) *Heart Disease: A Textbook of Cardiovascular Medicine*, Vol. 1, 6th edn, London, W.B. Saunders Co.
6. Brinker, J. A., Davidson, C. J. and Laskey, W. (2005) 'Preventing in-hospital cardiac and renal complications in high-risk PCI patients', *European Heart Journal Supplements*, **7** (Suppl G): G13–25, available online at *www.eurheartj/sui054*.
7. Carter, L. and Lamerton, M. (1996) 'Understanding balloon mitral valvuloplasty: The Inoue technique', *Intensive and Critical Care Nursing*, **12**: 147–54.
8. Cheng, T. O. (2000) 'The history of balloon valvuloplasty', *Journal of Interventional Cardiology*, **13**(5): 365–73.
9. Cheng, T. O. (2003) 'All roads lead to Rome: Transjugular or transfemoral approach to percutaneous transseptal balloon mitral valvuloplasty', *Catheterisation and Cardiovascular Intervention*, **59**: 266–7.

10. DVLA (2006) *For Medical Practitioners: At a Glance Guide to the Current Medical Standards of Fitness to Drive*, February, available online at *www.dvla.gov.uk*.
11. Galli, G. (2005) 'Ask the experts: Re removing arterial and venous sheaths after PCI', *Critical Care Nurse*, available online at *www.findarticles.com*.
12. Hughes, S. (2002) 'The effects of pre-operative information', *Nursing Standard*, **16**: 28, 33–7.
13. Julian, D. G., Cowan, J. C. and McLenachan, J. M. (2005) *Cardiology*, 8th edn, London, Elsevier Saunders.
14. Juran, N., Rouse, C., Smith, D., O'Brien, M., DeLuca, S. and Sigmon, K. (1999) 'Nursing interventions to decrease bleeding at the femoral access site after percutaneous coronary intervention', *American Journal of Critical Care*, **8**(5): 303–13.
15. Keeling, A., Fisher, C., Haugh, K., Powers, E. and Turner, M. (2000) 'Reducing time in bed after percutaneous transluminal coronary angioplasty (TIBS III)', *American Journal of Critical Care*, **9**(3): 185–7.
16. Kern, M. (2003) *The Cardiac Catheterisation Handbook*, 4th edn, London, Mosby.
17. Logemann, T., Luetmer, P., Kaliebe, J., Olson, K. and Murdock, D. (1999) 'Two versus six hours of bed rest following left-sided cardiac catheterisation and a meta-analysis of early ambulation trials', *The American Journal of Cardiology*, **84**: 486–8.
18. Matthews, R. (2004) 'Surgical management of aortic and mitral valve disease: An overview', *Professional Nurse*, **19**(5): 296–9.
19. Montalsecot, G., Andersen, H., Antoniucer, D., Betriu, A., de Boer, M., Grip, L., *et al.* (2004) 'Recommendations on percutaneous coronary intervention for the reperfusion of acute ST elevation myocardial infarction', *Heart*, 90, available online at *http://heart.bmjjournals.com/cgi/content/full/90/6/e37*.
20. Morton, P. G., Fontaine, D. K., Hudak, C. M. and Gallo, B. M. (2005) *Critical Care Nursing: A Holistic Approach*, 8th edn, Philadelphia, PA, Lippincott Williams & Wilkins.
21. Norell, M. and Perrins, J. (2003) *Essential Interventional Cardiology*, Philadelphia, PA, W.B. Saunders Co.
22. Nursing Midwifery Council (2002) *Guidelines for the Administration of Medicines*, London, Nursing Midwifery Council.
23. Sheppard, M. and Wright, M. (2000) *Principles and Practice of High Dependency Nursing*, Edinburgh, Bailliere Tindall.
24. Swanton, R. H. (2003) *Pocket Consultant Cardiology*, 5th edn, Oxford, Blackwell Publishing.
25. Thompson, P. (1997) *Coronary Care Manual*, London, Churchill Livingstone.
26. Topol, E. J. (1999) *Textbook of Interventional Cardiology*, 3rd edn, London, W.B. Saunders Co.
27. Tortora, G. J. and Derrickson, B. (2006) *Principles of Anatomy and Physiology*, 8th edn, Chichester, John Wiley and Sons Inc.
28. Woods, S., Froelicher, E. and Motzer, S. (2000) *Cardiac Nursing*, 4th edn, Philadelphia, PA, Lippincott Williams & Wilkins.

7 Atrial Septal Defect Closure

SEPTAL DEFECTS

Septal defects can be defined as abnormal communications between the left and right sides of the heart (23). They are more generally known as a 'hole in the heart'.

Septal defects are the most commonly occurring congenital cardiac defect seen in live births. About 3% of full-term babies have a ventricular septal defect (21), whilst atrial septal defects comprise 10% of all congenital heart anomalies (26).

The majority of congenital ventricular septal defects close spontaneously by the age of 1 year and pose few clinical problems (21). Patients with small ventricular septal defects usually live a normal lifespan, but they are exposed to the risk of infective endocarditis. They should be prescribed prophylactic antibiotics, when appropriate, such as prior to dental work, for example. However, large ventricular septal defects or those with multiple holes may lead to cardiac failure and will need surgical repair (10).

Atrial septal defects are classified by the portion of the atrial septum in which they occur. The presentation of symptoms and treatments available depends on where the defect is positioned in the atrial septum (23). Whilst the majority of septal defects present in childhood or early adolescence, patients with a secundum atrial septal defect are usually asymptomatic in childhood and may not be diagnosed until the patient is 40–50 years old (23). For this reason, those with a secundum atrial septal defect are one of the largest groups of patients with congenital heart disease seen by an adult cardiologist (21).

SECUNDUM ATRIAL SEPTAL DEFECT

A secundum atrial septal defect is one or more openings between the right atria and the left atria, but does not encroach on the atrioventricular valves (10) (see Figure 7.1). In the otherwise normal heart, secundum atrial septal defects cause a constant flow of blood from the left to the right across the defect, particularly on diastole. The shunt imparts a volume load on the right ventricle, causing dilation and progressive myocardial changes. This may contribute to the development of right heart failure in later life. Chronic atrial enlargement may cause atrial arrhythmias, usually atrial flutter or fibrillation, which are more common after the third decade of life and become more frequent with increasing age. The increased pulmonary blood flow exerts increased shear stress forces on the pulmonary

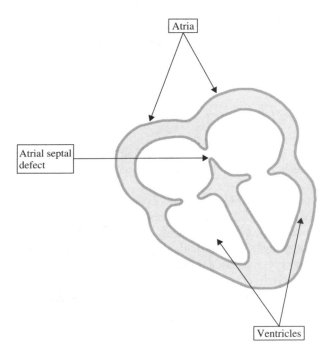

Figure 7.1. Atrial septal defect.

vascular bed, with subsequent dysfunction and morphological changes leading to pulmonary vascular disease (16).

In addition, late onset of mitral incompetency can occur, as can thrombosis of large pulmonary arteries. Therefore, any patients with a large atrial septal defect (ASD) (i.e. one that causes right-ventricular dilatation) need prophylactic closure, either surgically or by one of the catheter-inserted closure devices (21). A patient with a small atrial septal defect may be at risk of a paradoxical embolism. Closure of the atrial septal defect not only eliminates this risk, but it also increases the patient's exercise capacity (1). Although right-ventricular volume usually returns to normal or near normal levels after ASD closure, the atrium may remain enlarged. Therefore, closing an atrial septal defect in adults does not eliminate the increased long-term risk of developing atrial fibrillation (1).

TRANSCATHETER CLOSURE DEVICES

Transcatheter atrial septal defect occlusion was first attempted in 1976 by King and Mills, but reliable occlusion devices have only recently become available (18). From the late 1980s, through the mid-1990s, the button device and ASDOS were used extensively across Europe. In the 1990s, Angel wings – the first self-centring device – was developed. Nowadays, both ASDOS and Angel wings are out of clinical use because of the increased risk of cardiac perforation. Currently, the Amplatzer Septal Occluder, the Starflex Septal Occluder and the Helex are the most frequently used devices worldwide (1). Basically, the majority of the devices consist of conjoined discs or a disc and fixator, with the disc composed of synthetic fabrics and a metal skeleton. When extruded from the sheath, one of the discs overlies the secundum atrial septal defect on the left atrial side and the second disc is extruded in the right atrium, with both discs overlying the defect and occluding it. For successful delivery of the device, there needs to be a concentric rim of tissue around the defect, which will allow the device to be deployed without interfering with atrioventricular valve function, and sufficient margins to maintain position and prevent embolisation (16) (see Figure 7.2).

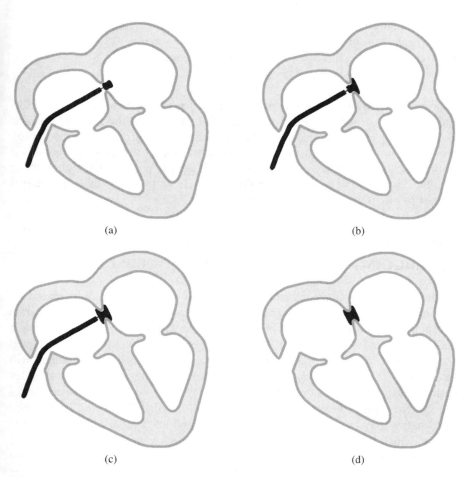

(a)   (b)

(c)   (d)

Figure 7.2. (a) Catheter delivering ASD device to the left atrium. (b) The distal disc is opened in the left atrium. (c) The proximal disc is opened in the right atrium by pulling the sheath back. (d) The device is released by unscrewing the wire.

The advent of transcatheter closure techniques for secundum atrial septal defects closure has minimised the degree of invasive surgery to the patient, with inherent advantages of almost no pain, discharge from the hospital the day after the procedure, and rapid recovery compared with heart surgery (16). It is now the method of choice, with a high success rate, low complication rate and applicability to all except small infants and neonates (18). However, the disadvantages associated with it are:

- suitable only for about 60% of atrial septal defects;
- risk of cerebral events (air or clot in the sheath);
- femoral vessel haemorrhage or occlusion;
- device embolisation may require surgical removal (and atrial septal defect repair) if transcatheter retrievals are not possible;
- mitral regurgitation;
- arrhythmias from atrial irritation in the first few weeks;
- atrial or aortic perforation (late) with some devices;
- residual shunt (18).

A possible disadvantage of the Amplatzer device is that it is somewhat bulky and consists of a large amount of nitinol. This has raised the issue of possible nickel toxicity in the future, although there have been no supporting data (16). Previously, the presence of more than one atrial septal defect was originally a contraindication to device closure; however, it is now possible to implant either a larger device to cover over the multiple defects or two devices if the defects are not in proximity to each other (18).

WHAT A PATIENT CAN EXPECT TO HAPPEN WHEN UNDERGOING ATRIAL SEPTAL DEFECT CLOSURE

As this is a percutaneous catheter procedure, the patient should be prepared for the procedure in a similar manner as that for a percutaneous coronary angiogram (Chapter 4). However, as transoesophageal echocardiography is used to assist the guidance and deployment of the device, this procedure is usually performed under general anaesthetic (18). Therefore, prior to the procedure, the patient will be assessed by an anaesthetist, who will take a detailed history, looking at issues such as past medical history, chronic illness, reaction to previous anaesthetics and current state of health (22). A combination of inhalational and intravenous anaesthetics may be used. Intravenous agents produce a rapid induction for the patient, which is more pleasant than breathing through a mask, whilst inhalational agents provide maintenance of anaesthesia. Although the inhalational agents are excreted through the lungs, allowing rapid emergence from unconsciousness, the intravenous agents need to be metabolised and excreted by the body, so patients may be drowsy when returning to the ward (22). The anaesthetist may prescribe a pre-medication to reduce anxiety and produce some sedation (14). These should be administered 45–70 minutes prior to the procedure, but only after the consent form has been signed, as they can make a patient drowsy (14).

Although there are a variety of atrial septal defect closure devices available, the method of implantation is similar with all devices (18). After anaesthetising the patient, transoesophageal echocardiography will be performed in order to assess the size and position of the defect and its anatomic relationship to the vena cava, aorta and atrioventricular valves, presence of additional defects and identification of all pulmonary veins (16).

Access to the femoral vessels is then performed by using the Seldinger technique – a 7–8 French sheath placed in the vein and a 4 French sheath in the artery for continuous blood pressure recording (16). Patients are then heparinised and a right-sided haemodynamic study will be performed, including shunt calculation (16).

The defect is accessed from a femoral vein and a stiff guidewire is placed in a left pulmonary vein. Over this wire, a sizing balloon catheter is advanced and inflated to occlude the defect. The size of the balloon that is just able to close the defect without excessive force is called the 'stretch' diameter of the defect and is used to select the correct device size. Accurate sizing is imperative to reduce the likelihood of device embolisation. An 8–12 French long sheath is advanced over the guidewire into the left atrium and meticulously de-aired. The chosen device is advanced and the distal (left atria) umbrella or disc is extruded into the left atrium. The sheath and device are withdrawn simultaneously to the atrial septum and, using fluoroscopy and transoesophageal echocardiography, the sheath is withdrawn further to deploy the proximal right atrial disc. The Amplatzer and ASDOS devices are completely retrievable and repositionable at this stage, the Cardioseal and Starflex devices can be retrieved (though not repositioned). Once the device appears to be correctly sited and stable, it is released. If the device is correctly sized, embolisation is uncommon. If embolisation does occur, transcatheter retrieval is not as easy as with the Rashkind ductal umbrella and surgical retrieval and atrial septal defect closure may be required (21). The delivery system and sheath can then be removed and pressure applied to the groin until bleeding is stopped (16).

If arterial catheterisation is necessary, for continuous blood pressure recording (16), administration of heparin is mandatory. Depending upon the amount of heparin used during the procedure, the patient may be warded with catheters in the insertion site (13). However, the delivery sheath and venous catheters are usually removed by the cardiologist, at the end of the procedure, whilst the patient is still in the cardiac laboratory or the recovery room (16). The cardiologist normally applies a few minutes' manual pressure over the puncture site until the femoral vein stops bleeding (13). A dressing may be applied or the patient may be asked to press gently on the puncture site.

POST PROCEDURE

Post-procedure care is similar to the routine for a percutaneous coronary angiogram (Chapter 4). The patient will be attached to a cardiac monitor, and the nurses will check the puncture site, pedal pulses and blood pressure half-hourly, while the patient is on bed rest, to observe for any complications, such as arrhythmias, vascular complications, systemic emboli and bleeding (18).

Depending on hospital protocol, the patient must continue complete bed rest for 4–6 hours after the sheath(s) has been removed (17). In order not to disturb the newly formed clot, patients should lie flat for the first 2 hours but they can sit up for the remaining time (12). Patients should be advised to keep the affected leg straight, and not move it too much during this time (8).

To prevent aspiration, the patient should be fully awake from the anaesthesia before they begin eating and drinking (22). Once they are awake, patients should be encouraged to drink plenty of fluid following the procedure in order to compensate for the diuretic action of the contrast dye, as well as to flush out the myocardial and vascular depressant drugs in their system, and to prevent hypotension. If the patient is unable to drink, intravenous fluids should be administered (1).

Patients normally remain in hospital overnight and are discharged on an anticoagulation regime to prevent thromboembolism from the device during endothelialisation (21). There is no consensus on what this anticoagulation regime should be. Many centres discharge patients home on aspirin alone, while others use a combination of aspirin, clopidogrel and warfarin (1). A small leak is common across the device in the first few days and months until it is fully endothelialised (18).

DISCHARGE ADVICE

As a prophylactic measure, patients should have antibiotics prior to any minor surgical procedures or dental work for 6–12 months after the procedure (1). Apart from this, discharge advice for atrial septal defect closure devices is similar to that of other percutaneous interventions that use heparin:

1. To feel the puncture site for signs of a growing lump over the next 2–3 days. If one develops or they get pins and needles in that leg, they should come back to their local hospital to have it scanned (26).
2. That they may get a bruise around the puncture site and normally this gets bigger as gravity pulls it down the leg. Unless it is painful, they should not worry about it.
3. That there may be a little bit of old dried blood or staining on their underwear. Again, this is nothing to worry about. If the blood is bright red and spurting, they should send for an ambulance. Whilst waiting for the ambulance, they should lie down on a firm surface and press firmly just above the puncture site.

4. Although it is very rare for problems like these to occur but in order to minimise them, they should:

- shower in preference to bathing for the next 2–3 days; if they only have a bath, they should use tepid water (26);
- not scrub vigorously over the puncture site;
- avoid heavy lifting and pulling for the next 2–3 days (26);
- note that the DVLA (2006) has no specific recommendations following an atrial septal defect repair. Therefore, it is recommended to follow the guidelines for an elective coronary angioplasty, which is to avoid driving for 1 week (7).

CARE PLANS

NURSING CONSIDERATION BEFORE THE PROCEDURE

The principle preparations for atrial septal defect closure are the same as those for any surgical procedure. The primary aim of nursing care is, therefore, to maximise patient safety and comfort during the procedure and optimise conditions for a successful outcome. This is achieved by ensuring that the patient is physically and psychologically prepared for the procedure, and that all documentation, including laboratory results and reports, are available to the cath lab staff (6).

PRE-PROCEDURE CARE PLAN FOR PATIENTS UNDERGOING AN ATRIAL SEPTAL DEFECT REPAIR

Action	Rationale
Obtain a brief history and check that biographical details and next of kin are correct	Checking the patient's biographical details and next of kin ensures that medical records are up-to-date and that in the event of an emergency, the correct person is contacted. Record keeping is a fundamental part of nursing care, ensuring high standards of clinical care and improving communication and dissemination of information (19)
Explain to the patient and their family what an atrial septal defect closure is and what will happen during and after the procedure. Provide an information booklet about the procedure	The period before an invasive procedure may be a time of anxiety and fear, for various reasons. Discussion and reassurance may help to relieve some of these feelings (9)

Action	Rationale
Check whether the patient is allergic to any food, drugs or other substances. Inform the doctor if the patient is allergic to any potential drugs used in the procedure	Patients with a history of allergy to iodine-containing substances, such as seafood or contrast agents, should be given an antihistamine and steroids before the procedure (26). In addition to this, a non-ionic contrast dye may be used for the procedure (4)
Check the medication regime. Metformin should be stopped 24 hours before the procedure	Metformin-associated lactic acidosis can be precipitated by the contrast dye used during the procedure. Although, in patients without renal failure, metformin can be used up to the day of contrast administration, ideally, it should be avoided 24 hours prior to the procedure (5; 23)
Nephrotoxic drugs and non-steroidal anti-inflammatory drugs should be avoided for a few days prior to the procedure	High doses of contrast dye may cause contrast-induced nephropathy. In order to minimise renal complications, it is advisable to avoid nephrotoxic drugs and non-steroidal anti-inflammatory drugs for several days prior to the procedure (5)
Warfarin should be stopped at least 48 hours prior to the procedure	Warfarin should be withheld for at least 48 hours prior to the procedure, to ensure an international normalised ratio (INR) of less than 2. Patients at high risk of thromboembolism should be admitted for heparinisation while the effects of oral anticoagulation wane (4)
Ideally, INR should be less than 2 (inform the cardiologist if it is higher)	Warfarin interferes with blood coagulation by blocking the effect of vitamin K. It has a long-acting half-life of 36–42 hours. The anticoagulation effect is described in a measurement of the INR. Therefore, any INR measurement of

Action	Rationale
	more than 2 increases the patient's risk of bleeding uncontrollably during and/or after the procedure (2)
Record blood pressure, pulse, temperature and blood glucose	This information should be evaluated to ensure that the patient is suitable for the procedure (4). It is also used to act as a baseline to compare the patient's vital signs with after the procedure (26)
Check for patent left and right pedal pulse	This information will be used for comparison in evaluating peripheral pulses after the catheterisation procedure (26)
Cannulate the patient	To provide intravenous access to administer prescribed drugs (13; 26)
If it is not against the patient's religious beliefs, ensure that the patient has shaved their groin appropriately	Body hair is removed in order to reduce infection risk during catheterisation (13; 26). Although most catheterisations are usually performed from the right femoral artery, it is expedient to routinely prepare both groins in case of difficulties in catheter advancement which may force a switch to the other groin once the procedure has begun (1)
Record the patient's height and weight	The dosage of anaesthesia is calculated on the patient's body mass index (18)
The patient should fast for at least 4–6 hours prior to the atrial septal defect closure	As the procedure will be performed under general anaesthesia, the patient needs to fast to reduce the risk of vomiting and aspirating fluid (18)
Remove dentures, artificial eyes, contact lenses and prosthetics	These items may cause confusion when the anaesthetist is assessing the unconscious patient (18)
Ensure that identification and allergy bands are correct, legible and secure	To ensure correct identification and prevent possible problems (26)

Action	Rationale
Encourage the patient to empty their bladder prior to taking the pre-medication	To help make them more comfortable (26)
Ensure that consent is obtained by the doctor performing the procedure	Consent for any procedure must be obtained by the doctor performing the procedure and a patient signature obtained. A full explanation of the procedure should be given, outlining the benefits and risks (18)
If the patient is a female of child-bearing age, she may be asked by the radiographer to sign a form indicating her pregnancy status	Pregnancy is a relative contraindicator in cardiac catheterisation procedures (13). However, as direct irradiation of the uterus can usually be avoided in procedures that involve structures above the diaphragm, fluoroscopic procedures on pregnant women may be justifiable in an emergency situation (1)

POST-PROCEDURE CARE PLAN

Goal/aim of care

The nursing care of patients following atrial septal defect closure is directed towards the prevention and detection of complications.

Action	Rationale
On warding, attach the patient to a cardiac monitor and check the following:	In order to observe the patient's vital signs post procedure (17)
Pulse	The pulse should be observed, as a mild sinus tachycardia (100–120 beats per minute) is not unusual after a catheterisation procedure. This may be a sign of anxiety, an indication of fluid loss due to diuresis or a reaction to medication used during the procedure. Fluids, time and reassurance often bring the

Action	Rationale
	heart rate down to more normal levels. Heart rates above 120 beats per minute should be evaluated for other causes, such as haemorrhage, more severe fluid imbalance, fever or arrhythmias. If not on betablockers, a bradycardia may indicate a vasovagal response, arrhythmias or an infarction and should be assessed by an electrocardiogram and correlated with other clinical signs, such as pain and blood pressure (26)
Blood pressure	Patients may return to the ward with a low blood pressure caused by drugs, such as vasodilators, administered during the procedure. In addition, the contrast dye acts as an osmotic diuretic and patients may become hypotensive due to volume depletion. Patients are thus kept on bed rest until fluid balance is restored, with oral liquids or by intravenous replacement. If the blood pressure is less than 75–80% of baseline, other causes such as blood loss or arrhythmias must be considered and assessed, and the doctor notified (26)
Pulse oximetry	Hypoxia occurs for a variety of reasons following anaesthesia. The administration of supplemental oxygen in the immediate post-operative phase will help to reduce the risk of hypoxia occurring. The aim is to maintain normal levels of arterial blood gases and peripheral oxygen saturations (22)
Respiratory rate	Anaesthesia and opiates may depress respiration. Although the anaesthetist aims to have reversed these effects

Action	Rationale
	by the time the patient is warded, there is potential for severe respiratory depression to be present in the immediate post-procedure period (22)
Pedal pulse	The most frequent complication of a percutaneous procedure is arterial thrombosis. The puncture site in the groin should be checked for visible bleeding, swelling or tenderness. The arterial pulse at the site and at points distal to it should be compared with pulses on the opposite limb and those recorded before the procedure. Capillary filling and the warmth of the limb should also be evaluated. Blanching, cramping, coolness, pain, numbness or tingling may indicate reduced perfusion and must be carefully evaluated. A diminished or absent pulse is a sign of serious arterial occlusion (13; 26). If a compression device is being used to achieve haemostasis, the pressure should be reduced. If this does not improve circulation, medical staff should be informed (26)
Check the puncture site for signs of bleeding or haematoma	Research shows that the majority of bleeding/haematoma was detected by nurses checking the groin (3)
Until the patient is mobile, check these observations half-hourly and ask the patient to report any feelings of wetness, stickiness, warmth or bleeding in the puncture-site area	Research shows that a large proportion of puncture-site bleeding was detected through the patient's calling for assistance (3)
Advise the patient to keep the affected leg straight whilst on bed rest	Bleeding and haematoma formation may occur when a patient moves the limb too vigorously (13; 26)

Action	Rationale
If the patient is a diabetic, check their blood sugar on warding	To ensure that the patient is not hypoglycaemic, as they may have fasted for long periods prior to the procedure (26)
Advise patients to inform the nurse if they experience any chest pain	Chest pain may indicate potential cardiac complications; therefore, nurses should be aware of it if it is present (17)
Ensure that any intravenous fluids are running at the correct rate, and administer any drugs prescribed post procedure	It is the ward nurses' responsibility to ensure that the prescribed drugs, intravenous or oral, are administered correctly (17; 20)
If the patient still has the femoral sheaths in situ, they can sit up at a 30° angle until the femoral sheaths are removed	Research has shown that no difference in bleeding at the catheter insertion site was observed whether the patient was lying flat or if the bed head was elevated by 30° (8; 11; 18)
Ensure that the patient is fully awake before providing them with something to eat or drink	During anaesthesia, voluntary muscular control is temporarily lost; therefore, post procedure, if the patient is not fully awake, fluids may be inhaled accidentally (22). Initially, try patients with sips of water
Observe urine output, as a poor urine output may be the first indication of contrast-induced renal failure	Contrast nephropathy is a recognised complication of procedures that use contrast dye (5) and a poor urine output is an early indication of this condition (13). However, as the contrast dye acts as an osmotic diuretic, patients may have an increase in urine output for a short time after the procedure (26)
If a vascular closure device was used to achieve haemostasis, such as an AngioSeal, please follow the manufacturer's guidelines about bed rest and mobilising the patient	Although these devices have been shown to reduce the time to obtain haemostasis (1; 13), the patient maintains the risk of developing cardiac complications such as

Action	Rationale
	bradycardia or hypotension as a result of the drugs used during the procedure (26); therefore, it is good policy to maintain cardiac monitoring for at least 4 hours after the procedure
If the patient has the introducer sheath still in the femoral artery, it should be removed as per hospital protocol or the cardiologist's advice	Femoral sheaths are normally removed 3–4 hours after catheterisation procedures that utilised heparin, to allow time for the heparin to dissipate (17; 18)
After the femoral sheath has been removed from the femoral artery and haemostasis has been achieved, the patient should remain on bed rest as per hospital protocol	Patients are advised to remain on bed rest in order not to disturb the newly formed clot over the puncture site. However, bed-rest post-sheath removal guidelines vary from hospital to hospital (12; 24). Keeling *et al.* (2000) suggest that lying the patient flat for 2 hours and then sitting them up for 2 hours is usually sufficient to ensure haemostasis (12). However, smaller studies since then indicate that it may be safe to reduce bed rest further (24)
Whilst on bed rest, advise patients to press on the puncture site if they cough or sneeze	Patients are advised to press on the puncture site while coughing or sneezing in order to prevent the newly formed clot from being disturbed (3)
Once mobile, pedal pulse and puncture-site observations may cease, unless the patient complains of numbness, pins and needles or a lump in the groin area or the puncture site begins to bleed	Complications such as bleeding or haematomas are normally observed within 10 minutes of ambulation (15)
Advise patients to take things slowly when they first mobilise	A patient may drop their blood pressure by simply standing up abruptly after prolonged bed rest (25)

Action	Rationale
Prior to discharge, the patient should be instructed about puncture-site care, and informed of any signs and symptoms which require a doctor's review. A discharge leaflet should be provided	So that patients will be aware of potential complications post discharge and know what to do in the event of these occurring (13)
Any changes in medication should be discussed with the patient	When discharging a patient, it is the nurses' responsibility to inform the patient about the medication that they have been prescribed so that they will take it correctly at home (20)
If the patient normally takes metformin, they should be advised to have their urea and electrolytes checked by their family doctor 48 hours after the procedure and restart it when advised to by them	Metformin is contraindicated in patients with renal dysfunction, as determined by elevated serum creatinine levels. Therefore, metformin should only be resumed after the renal function is found to be normal (18)

REFERENCES

1. Baim, D. S. (2006) *Grossman's Cardiac Catheterisation: Angiography and Intervention*, 7th edn, Philadelphia, PA, Lippincott Williams & Wilkins.
2. Blann, A., Landray, M. and Lip, G. (2002) 'An overview of antithrombotic therapy', *British Medical Journal*, **325**: 762–5.
3. Botti, M., Williamson, B. and Steen, K. (2001) 'Coronary angiography observations: Evidence-based or ritualistic practice?', *Heart & Lung: The Journal of Acute and Critical Care*, **30**(2): 138–45.
4. Braunweld, E., Zipes, D. and Libby, P. (2001) *Heart Disease: A Textbook of Cardiovascular Medicine*, Vol. 1, 6th edn, London, W.B. Saunders Co.
5. Brinker, J. A., Davidson, C. J. and Laskey, W. (2005) 'Preventing in-hospital cardiac and renal complications in high-risk PCI patients', *European Heart Journal Supplements*, **7**(Suppl G): G13–25, available online at *www.eurheartj/sui054*.
6. Carter, L. and Lamerton, M. (1996) 'Understanding balloon mitral valvuloplasty: The Inoue technique', *Intensive and Critical Care Nursing*, **12**: 147–54.
7. DVLA (2006) *For Medical Practitioners: At a Glance Guide to the Current Medical Standards of Fitness to Drive*, February, available online at *www.dvla.gov.uk*.
8. Galli, G. (2005) 'Ask the experts: Re removing arterial and venous sheaths after PCI', *Critical Care Nurse*, available online at *www.findarticles.com*.
9. Hughes, S. (2002) 'The effects of pre-operative information', *Nursing Standard*, **16**: 28, 33–7.

10. Julian, D. G., Cowan, J. C. and McLenachan, J. M. (2005) *Cardiology*, 8th edn, London, Elsevier Saunders.
11. Juran, N., Rouse, C., Smith, D., O'Brien, M., DeLuca, S. and Sigmon, K. (1999) 'Nursing interventions to decrease bleeding at the femoral access site after percutaneous coronary intervention', *American Journal of Critical Care*, **8**(5): 303–13.
12. Keeling, A., Fisher, C., Haugh, K., Powers, E. and Turner, M. (2000) 'Reducing time in bed after percutaneous transluminal coronary angioplasty (TIBS III)', *American Journal of Critical Care*, **9**(3): 185–7.
13. Kern, M. (2003) *The Cardiac Catheterisation Handbook*, 4th edn, London, Mosby.
14. Lemone, P. and Burke, K. (2004) *Medical/Surgical Nursing: Critical Thinking in Client Care*, 3rd edn, Upper Saddle River, NJ, Pearson Prentice Hall.
15. Logemann, T., Luetmer, P., Kaliebe, J., Olson, K. and Murdock, D. (1999) 'Two versus six hours of bed rest following left-sided cardiac catheterisation and a meta-analysis of early ambulation trials', *The American Journal of Cardiology*, **84**: 486–8.
16. Matitiau, A., Birk, E., Kachko, L., Blieden, L. C. and Bruckheimer, E. (2001) 'Transcatheter closure of secundum atrial septal defects with the Amplatzer occluder early experience', *IMAJ*, **3**(Jan): 32–5.
17. Morton, P. G., Fontaine, D. K., Hudak, C. M. and Gallo, B. M. (2005) *Critical Care Nursing: A Holistic Approach*, 8th edn, Philadelphia, PA, Lippincott Williams & Wilkins.
18. Norell, M. and Perrins, J. (2003) *Essential Interventional Cardiology*, Philadelphia, PA, W.B. Saunders Co.
19. Nursing Midwifery Council (2002a) *Guidelines for Records and Record Keeping*, London, Nursing and Midwifery Council, April.
20. Nursing Midwifery Council (2002b) *Guidelines for the Administration of Medicines*, London, Nursing and Midwifery Council.
21. Rosendorff, C. (2005) *Essential Cardiology: Principles and Practice*, 2nd edn, Totowa, NJ, Humana Press.
22. Sheppard, M. and Wright, M. (2000) *Principles and Practice of High Dependency Nursing*, Edinburgh, Bailliere Tindall.
23. Swanton, R. H. (2003) *Cardiology*, 3rd edn, Malden, MA, Blackwell Publishing.
24. Tagney, J. and Lackie, D. (2005) 'Bed-rest post-femoral arterial sheath removal: What is safe practice? A clinical audit', *British Association of Critical Care Nurses, Nursing in Critical Care*, **10**(4): 167–73.
25. Topol, E. J. (1999) *Textbook of Interventional Cardiology*, 3rd edn, London, W.B. Saunders Co.
26. Woods, S., Froelicher, E. and Motzer, S. (2000) *Cardiac Nursing*, 4th edn, Philadelphia, PA, Lippincott Williams & Wilkins.

8 Electrophysiology Studies and Radio-Frequency Ablation

NORMAL HEART BEAT

The heart has a natural electrical system which makes it beat at a regular rhythm (Figure 8.1). High in the right atrium, there is a cluster of self-exciting cells called the sinoatrial node (SA node). This acts as a natural pacemaker, which produces regular electrical impulses that spread across both atria causing them to contract simultaneously and squeeze the blood into the ventricles (Figure 8.2). In a normal heart, there is only one electrical connection between the atria and the ventricles. This is called the atrioventricular node (AV node) and is located in the lower right atria. While the atria are contracting, the electrical impulse is slowed, as it passes through the AV node to the bundle of His and the Purkinje fibres. These provide the conduction pathway along which the electrical impulse travels through the ventricles, causing them to contract simultaneously and squeeze the blood out to the lungs and the body (22; 29).

ABNORMAL HEARTBEATS

Changes in the heart's electrical system can cause periodic episodes of an abnormal heart rhythm. When this occurs, the heart can beat very rapidly and cause

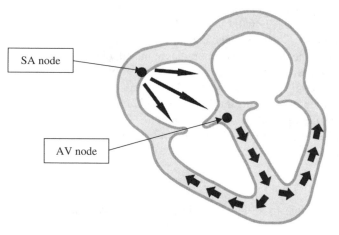

Figure 8.1. Normal conduction sinus rhythm.

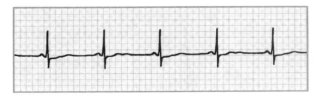

Figure 8.2. ECG strip showing sinus rhythm.

symptoms of palpitations, light-headedness or dizziness, shortness of breath, a feeling of fullness in the throat, chest pain/pressure, fatigue or fainting (22). These signs and symptoms can be disabling, and may disrupt patients' daily activities because they may occur at unpredictable times and last from minutes to hours (1). In addition, patients with cardiac arrhythmias may experience life-threatening signs and symptoms of cardiac arrest (1).

The most common type of arrhythmia is fast heart rhythms that originate in the atria. They are referred to as 'supraventricular tachycardia', or 'SVT' (as they occur above the ventricles). These arrhythmias are generally considered benign and are not life-threatening. There are five major types of rhythm disturbances that arise in the atria:

1. atrial fibrillation;
2. atrial flutter;
3. AV nodal re-entrant tachycardia;
4. AV reciprocating tachycardia; and
5. atrial tachycardia (22).

ATRIAL FIBRILLATION

Atrial fibrillation (AF) is the most common sustained tachyarrhythmia, and generally occurs in people with underlying heart disease (Figure 8.3). Atrial fibrillation can also occur in people without other heart problems – a condition termed 'lone atrial fibrillation'. The exact mechanism of AF is still being investigated. In some patients, it may be due to wandering, disorganised, electrical circuits (wavefronts) throughout the atria. In others, it may be caused by a single, rapidly firing electrical spot (focus), which is commonly located in one of the pulmonary veins near where they empty into the left atrium (22).

During atrial fibrillation, the AV node is bombarded with many electrical impulses from the atria (the abnormal wavefronts), which may cause the ventricles to beat rapidly and irregularly (22).

ATRIAL FLUTTER

Atrial flutter is due to an electrical impulse that travels around a defined circuit in the right atrium. This impulse is funnelled through a small region of heart tissue (isthmus) located at the bottom of the right atrium (22) (Figure 8.4).

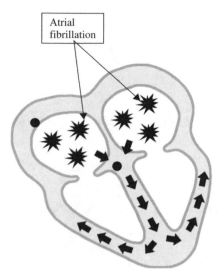

Figure 8.3. Atrial fibrillation.

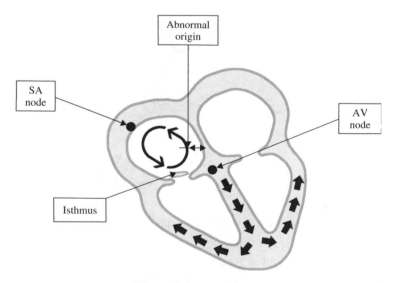

Figure 8.4. Atrial flutter.

Atrial fibrillation and atrial flutter are usually easily identified, as they have a characteristic appearance on the electrocardiogram (ECG) (Figures 8.5 and 8.6). The other three SVTs are often harder to distinguish on an ECG (22).

Of these, the most common is 'AV nodal re-entrant tachycardia' (AVNRT) and originates in the area of the AV node (Figure 8.7). Apart from atrial fibrillation, this mechanism accounts for approximately 60% of all SVTs. Some people are

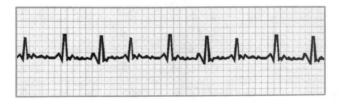

Figure 8.5. ECG strip showing atrial fibrillation.

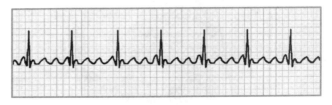

Figure 8.6. ECG strip of atrial flutter.

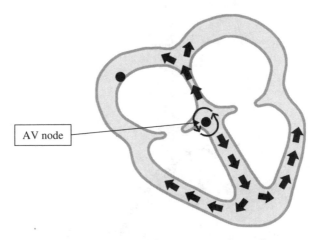

Figure 8.7. AV nodal re-entrant tachycardia.

born with two pathways within their AV node (22), usually consisting of a fast pathway and a slow pathway. The AVNRT is initiated when a premature beat from the atrium is blocked in the fast pathway. The early beat conducts down the slow pathway. It then re-enters back up the slow pathway, causing a rapid heart beat (22; 30).

Some people are born with an extra connection (accessory pathway) between the atria and the ventricles. When the accessory pathway is visible on the electrocardiogram (ECG), this is called the 'Wolff–Parkinson–White' syndrome, or 'WPW'. Other people may have an accessory pathway which is not visible. This is called a 'concealed' (or hidden) accessory pathway. Under the right conditions,

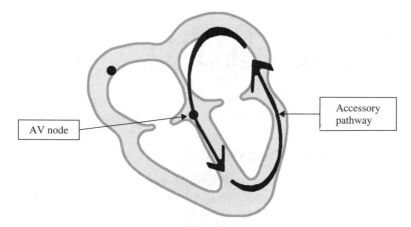

Figure 8.8. AV reciprocating tachycardia.

an electrical impulse can travel down the normal electrical connection and then back up the accessory pathway, causing a rapid heart beat. This is known as 'AV reciprocating tachycardia' (AVRT) (Figure 8.8). This mechanism accounts for approximately 30% of SVTs (22).

If atrial fibrillation occurs in a patient with WPW, a life-threatening situation may develop if conduction over the accessory pathway is rapid enough to induce ventricular fibrillation (30).

ATRIAL TACHYCARDIA

Atrial tachycardia may be due to an abnormal electrical impulse originating from a spot (focus) in the atria other than the normal pacemaker centre (SA node) (22) (Figures 8.9 and 8.10). Focal atria tachycardia is the least common form of SVT (21).

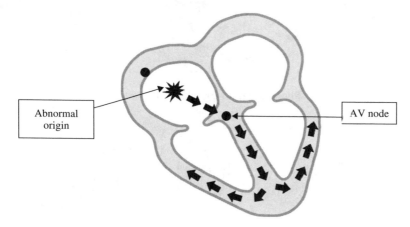

Figure 8.9. Atrial tachycardia.

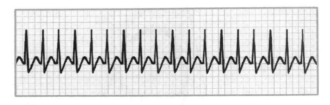

Figure 8.10. ECG strip of atrial tachycardia.

VENTRICULAR ARRHYTHMIAS

Heart rhythm disturbances can also originate in the ventricles, the most common being ventricular tachycardia (VT) (Figure 8.11). Ventricular arrhythmias tend to be more serious than supraventricular arrhythmias and are generally life-threatening. VT most often arises from areas of scar tissue in the ventricle, which is the result of a heart attack. However, VT can also occur in a normal, healthy heart (22).

Because sustained arrhythmias are often episodic in nature or can terminate spontaneously, it can be difficult to record them on conventional ECG recordings (28) (Figure 8.12). The use of Holter monitors and reveal devices can assist

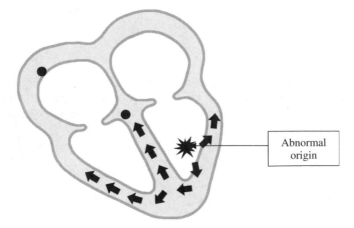

Figure 8.11. Ventricular tachycardia.

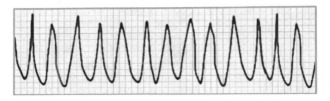

Figure 8.12. ECG strip of ventricular tachycardia.

in capturing these arrhythmias. However, it can still be difficult to differentiate between some arrhythmias, such as ventricular tachycardia and supraventricular tachycardia, from ECG recordings alone (12). The emergence in the 1970s of a new invasive procedure known as electrophysiology studies (EPSs) has improved arrhythmia diagnosis (14).

WHAT ARE ELECTROPHYSIOLOGY STUDIES?

Electrophysiology studies are able to localise and record the electrical activity of specific sections of the conduction system, as well as induce arrhythmias for evaluation (1). Although EPSs were used primarily for diagnostic purposes, the indications and applications of EPS have expanded greatly since the late 1990s (14).

Nowadays, EPSs are used for:

- arrhythmia diagnosis;
- assessing the efficacy of antiarrhythmic drugs;
- assessing the patient's predisposition for spontaneously occurring arrhythmias;
- distinguishing between a supraventricular rhythm and ventricular tachycardia;
- identifying the origin of a ventricular arrhythmia or the site of a bypass tract;
- evaluating the need for and efficacy of an automated implantable cardioverter defibrillator (AICD);
- performing pre-ablation mapping (14; 28; 29).

The electrophysiology study either may be performed for diagnostic purposes only or may be part of a combined diagnostic and therapeutic (e.g. ablation) procedure (28). Nowadays, if the EPS is just a diagnostic study, the patient may be able to go home the same day, once bleeding at the puncture sites has stopped (7).

An electrophysiology study is performed under sterile conditions in a laboratory, similarly to a cardiac catheterisation. Fluoroscopy is used to guide custom-designed electrodes into appropriate positions. Different parts of the heart are accessible by different veins (and arteries); therefore, in order for the electrodes to reach the desired location in the heart, catheters are usually introduced percutaneously via the appropriate vein for that location. The femoral, brachial or basilic veins are normally used for access. However, the subclavian and jugular veins may also be used. Arterial cannulation is performed only if left-ventricular stimulation is necessary (1).

The electrodes are placed in a juxtaposition to several sites in the atria, ventricles and also adjacent to the bundle of His (12). The electrical recording from these different locations in the heart and the response to electrical stimulation via the electrodes allow detailed information about the cause of the arrhythmias to be identified. A potentially important part of an electrophysiology study is the use of intracardiac recordings to determine activation sequences during arrhythmias. This process is usually called 'mapping'. Analyses of the responses of an arrhythmia to various pacing techniques are also components of the mapping process (28).

Once an arrhythmia has been identified, the next step is to choose the most effective treatment regimen (29). Before commencing a patient on therapy with an antiarrhythmic drug, it is essential to consider the advantages and disadvantages of the drug treatment. As a group, antiarrhythmic drugs have the potential to do harm as well as good. It is well established that under some circumstances, antiarrhythmic drugs may exacerbate existing arrhythmias or even create new ones (12). However, in the 1980s, the introduction of catheter ablation revolutionised the treatment of arrhythmias (28).

WHAT IS RADIO-FREQUENCY ABLATION?

Catheter ablation is an interventional discipline within electrophysiology whereby an arrhythmogenic focus or critical portion of an arrhythmia circuit is identified, localised and subsequently destroyed by means of a percutaneous transcatheter technique (14). Ablation using direct current shocks was first employed for the treatment of human cardiac arrhythmias in 1982. After it had been demonstrated that atrioventricular conduction could be permanently interrupted, the technique was applied to a variety of re-entrant and ectopic arrhythmias (26).

Introduced in 1987, radiofrequency has replaced direct current shock energy because of its relative ease of use, the smaller homogeneous lesions it produces and its greater safety (26). Radio-frequency current uses energy similar to surgical diathermy. The use of this form of energy is a huge advance and at last has brought a permanent non-surgical cure to many patients with disabling tachycardias whose lives were a misery on drug treatment. Particular advantages of the technique are:

- low voltages only required (40–60 V), no cardiac barotraumas;
- no neuromuscular stimulation, so no general anaesthetic required, sedation only;
- discrete, precise lesions with minimal cardiac damage;
- possible to perform electrophysiological study and ablation in one procedure;
- high success rate and low recurrence rate, with very few complications (24).

The disadvantage with the technique is that it is time-consuming, with a long learning curve and often a long screening time. The average length of the procedure is 1–3 hours, but occasionally more than 6 hours, with screening times of 2 hours (24).

Usually, diagnostic electrophysiological testing and radio-frequency ablation are accomplished in a single procedure. This combined approach not only enhances the efficiency of treatment, but also results in substantially decreased costs when compared with other therapeutic modalities (7).

The ablating catheter tip must be negotiated gradually to within less than 1 mm of the accessory pathway or arrhythmogenic focus (24). Then, the radio-frequency current is passed down an electrode catheter positioned in contact with the endocardium, producing a small area of thermal tissue destruction (12). Sometimes, multiple accessory pathways have to be dealt with. Ablation can, if necessary, be performed in the coronary sinus but there is a small risk of pericarditis or perforation here (24).

Radio-frequency ablation has become the first line of therapy, as it is safe and cost-effective and eliminates the underlying arrhythmia mechanism with minimal risk of complications. The majority (95%) of patients go home the day after catheter ablation (21).

COMPLICATIONS OF ELECTROPHYSIOLOGY STUDIES AND RADIO-FREQUENCY ABLATION

Several studies found that the mortality associated with EPS/radio-frequency ablation is extremely low, ranging from 0.08 to 0.2% (4). Complications of the procedure are usually associated with catheterisation and catheter manipulation rather than stimulation and the induction of arrhythmias (14). Complications resulting from catheterisation include haematomas, deep vein thrombosis. arterial perforation and arteriovenous fistula. If the subclavian or internal jugular venous approaches are used, haemothorax and pneumothorax are recognised potential complications (14). Catheter manipulation may cause valvular damage, micro emboli, perforation of the coronary sinus or myocardial wall, coronary artery dissection and thrombosis (4). The delivery of the radio-frequency energy may cause AV block, myocardial perforation, coronary artery spasm or occlusion, transient ischaemic attacks and cerebrovascular accidents (4). Although it is a small risk, ranging from 0.17 to 1.0% (4), if the AV node is destroyed, it will result in complete heart block and the patient may need permanent pacing (14). Including all these potential complications, the overall complication rates remain low and range from 1.82 to 4.4%, depending on which study you read (4).

WHAT A PATIENT CAN EXPECT WHEN UNDERGOING AN ELECTROPHYSIOLOGY STUDY/RADIO-FREQUENCY ABLATION

PRIOR TO ADMISSION

The results of the EPS must be analysed in the context of the patient's clinical presentation and cardiac substrate. All reversible causes of arrhythmias (e.g. ischaemia, electrolyte imbalance) will be ruled out (1). The cardiologist performing the procedure must comprehensively evaluate the patient before the EPS

Table 8.1. Evaluation before the electrophysiologic testing

Procedure	Purpose
History and physical examination	Identify signs and symptoms of cardiac or neurologic disease Identify factors known to exacerbate arrhythmias Determine details of syncopal events
Neurological evaluation (if history and physical suggest)	Rule out seizure disorder
Electroencephalogram Computed topography/magnetic resonance imaging Carotid ultrasound	Identify focal lesion Identify significant cerebrovascular disease
12-lead ECG	Identify previous myocardial infarction Identify intra-ventricular conduction delays Identify prolonged QT interval Identify pre-excitation syndromes
Event recorder	Correlation symptoms with ECG events
Head-up tilt table testing	Diagnose vasovagal/vasodepressor syncope
Echocardiogram and radio nucleotide ventriculography	Assessment of left-ventricular and right-ventricular size and function
Stress test (with or without perfusion scanning)	Detection of reversible ischaemia
	Assessment of effects of catecholamines on arrhythmia induction
Cardiac catheterisation	Definition of coronary anatomy

Reprinted with permission from Kern (2003) p. 334. Elsevier, London.

and plan the procedure based on the information being sought in the individual patient. Wherever possible, ECG documentation of the arrhythmia – preferably a 12-lead ECG – should be obtained and the patient may undergo some or all of the procedures listed in Table 8.1 (14).

PREPARING A PATIENT FOR AN ELECTROPHYSIOLOGY STUDY/RADIO-FREQUENCY ABLATION

As this is a percutaneous catheter procedure, the patient should be prepared for the procedure in a similar manner as that for a percutaneous coronary angiogram (Chapter 4). However, prior to coming into hospital, patients should be advised to:

- Discontinue all antiarrhythmic medications at least five half-lives before the day of the procedure (1; 14). This is in order to study the arrhythmias without the influence of any antiarrhythmic drugs (29). The patient may continue taking other medication in order to prevent haemodynamic compromise (1), apart from warfarin.
- Fast for at least 4–6 hours prior to the procedure. However, a small amount of water can be taken with essential medications. This is due to the patient's possibly requiring sedation and cardioversion to terminate arrhythmia (1).
- Shave both groin areas. A nurse can assist with this if the patient has any difficulties (29).

In order to help to reduce anxiety, the nurse should provide information about the EPS/radio-frequency procedure to the patient and their families in a simple and concise format, and in an empathetic manner (1). In addition to having what the procedure entails explained to them, the patients should be informed that they may feel sensations similar to their palpitations during the EPS, if the cardiologist triggers their arrhythmia (1). Depending on consultant preference, an ECG and urea and electrolytes should be checked on the morning of the procedure (14).

DURING THE ELECTROPHYSIOLOGY STUDY/ABLATION

Electrophysiology studies/radio-frequency ablations are performed while the patient is awake. Occasionally, sedation will be used if the patient is unusually anxious, but since patient cooperation and verbal response to stimulation are extremely helpful to the study, heavy sedation is undesirable (29).

A routine initial diagnostic EPS usually involves insertion of at least three catheters, most commonly via the femoral veins. These large veins easily permit the introduction of two 5–7 French catheters per vein. The number of catheters required and venous access selected depend on the type of study being performed and the data being collected (14). However, in order to reach certain parts of the heart, the subclavian vein, jugular vein or femoral artery may be used (24). In addition, an arterial line may be inserted in patients with suspected ventricular tachycardia or fibrillation, to monitor blood pressure (29).

The selected insertion sites are usually anaesthetised with a local anaesthetic such as lignocaine. Therefore, the patient should not feel any pain during the procedure but may feel some pressure sensation during sheath insertion. However, they may feel a stinging sensation when the anaesthetic is being injected (1).

On arrival at the cardiac laboratory, surface ECG leads are placed on the chest so that simultaneous recordings can be made (1; 29). A variety of electrode catheters can be used to perform an EPS. Multi-polar catheters are positioned in the heart under fluoroscopy. Once the patient has been prepared properly and the catheters are placed, a baseline EPS is undertaken to document the properties of the arrhythmia and the inducibility of the arrhythmia. After the characteristics of the arrhythmia have been evaluated fully, the mapping and ablation procedures are begun (14).

When the optimal site for an ablation has been localised, the radio-frequency current is applied to the distal pole of the mapping catheter. Typically, 15–35 W of current is applied over 30–60 seconds to achieve a target temperature of 60 °C, while the rhythm and intracardiac electrograms are monitored closely (14). In many laboratories, prophylactic broad-spectrum intravenous antibiotics are administered before and during the ablation (14).

After the ablation, there is typically a 15–30-minute waiting period, during which repeat EPS is undertaken. This EPS is used to document the successful ablation or signs of early recurrence. If no evidence of recurrent tachycardia is seen during approximately 30 minutes after ablation, the procedure can be terminated and the patient returned to their hospital room (14).

If arterial catheterisation is necessary, administration of heparin is mandatory. Patients undergoing prolonged studies involving venous access or with a history of venous thromboembolism should also receive heparin (14). Depending upon the amount of heparin used during the procedure, the patient may be warded with catheters in the insertion site. However, the percutaneous venous catheters are usually removed by the cardiologist at the end of the procedure, whilst the patient is still in the cardiac laboratory or the recovery room. The cardiologist normally applies a few minutes' manual pressure over the puncture site until the bleeding has stopped (14). A dressing may be applied or the patient may be asked to press gently on the puncture site.

POST ELECTROPHYSIOLOGY STUDY/RADIO-FREQUENCY ABLATION

On warding the patient, the nurse should check the catheter site for bleeding, swelling or diminished circulation to the distal extremities. If blood is seen on the dressing, place a new, firm-pressure dressing on the site and check as appropriate for the patient – but at least every 15 minutes, for a period of 1 hour. Remind the patient of the importance of keeping the extremity straight for the prescribed time (29). Depending on the cardiologist, they are recommended to keep the leg straight for 1–2 hours to allow the venous puncture to heal and for 2–4 hours if the femoral artery was punctured. Although the patient is allowed to mobilise after the prescribed bed-rest time is completed, the patient should be observed with cardiac monitoring overnight. During this time, early recurrence can be detected or iatrogenic conduction abnormalities observed (14; 26).

The patient should be observed for other complications that can result from the procedure, such as pneumothorax, the development of post-procedure fever or vascular-associated injury associated with the catheterisation procedure (14). One potential problem that can occur during an EPS is the development of a vaso-vagal reaction with either catheter insertion or withdrawal. Pallor, diaphoresis, nausea, vomiting, dizziness, bradycardia or hypotension can result from vagal stimulation (29).

Additionally, a rare complication is the development of a pericardial effusion resulting from a small ventricular puncture. Small leaks usually repair themselves without complication. However, a rapid leaking of blood into the pericardial sac can result in cardiac tamponade. Symptoms associated with this include pallor, hypotension, sweating, loss of voltage on ECG and chest pain. The pericardial sac must be decompressed to restore adequate cardiac output. In general, complications following EPSs are very rare (29).

If antiarrhythmic drug trials are performed, the patient's response to therapy is assessed by measuring vital signs, any ECG changes, side effects of the drug and the efficacy of the drug in controlling the patient's rhythm (29). Monitoring for tachyarrhythmias and/or side effects from the new drug is very important. Therefore, nurses should document any further episodes of arrhythmias. Allowing patients to verbalise fears and anxieties about future studies, impending surgery or the need for long-term antiarrhythmic drug therapy promotes comfort and aids compliance with the treatment regimen. Slow, deep breathing and relaxation techniques may be helpful in reducing anxiety (1; 29).

Following radio-frequency ablation, the patient is kept in overnight and echocardiography may be performed the following morning, before discharge, to exclude a possible pericardial collection (24). It is good practice to record an ECG the following morning, to check that the arrhythmia has not recurred or that the AV node has not been damaged, by checking the P–R interval (7).

Depending on the cardiologist, prophylactic antibiotics may be prescribed for 3 days post ablation to prevent endocarditis and aspirin is administered for 1 month post ablation to prevent blood clots' forming on the ablation area (7).

Doses may vary, depending on the consultant (10).

DISCHARGE ADVICE

Although the patient can typically be discharged the morning after the procedure with few physical limitations (14), the patient should be advised:

1. To feel the puncture site for signs of a growing lump over the next 2–3 days. If one develops or they get pins and needles in that leg, they should come back to their local hospital to have it scanned.
2. That they may get a bruise around the puncture site and normally this gets bigger as gravity pulls it down the leg. Unless it is painful, they should not worry about this.
3. That there may a little bit of blood staining on their underwear. If the blood is bright red and spurting, they should send for an ambulance. Whilst waiting

for the ambulance, they should lie down on a firm surface and press firmly just above the puncture site (10).

4. Although it is rare for such complications to occur, in order to minimise them, it is recommended that for a few days following the procedure, they should:
   - avoid heavy lifting for 2–3 days (10);
   - shower in preference to bathing but if they only have a bath, use lukewarm water (30);
   - not rub hard over the puncture site – pat it gently;
   - note that the DVLA (2006) recommends no driving for 1 week after a successful ablation. Group 2 licence holders (lorries/buses) are disqualified from driving for 6 weeks. If they hold a professional licence, they should advise the DVLA that they have had a catheter ablation, otherwise they do not need to inform them (9).

CARE PLANS

PRE-PROCEDURE CARE PLAN: NURSING CONSIDERATION BEFORE THE PROCEDURE

The principle preparations for EPS/radio-frequency ablation are the same as for any catheterisation procedure (30). The primary aim of nursing care is, therefore, to maximise patient safety and comfort during the procedure and optimise conditions for a successful outcome. This is achieved by ensuring that the patient is physically and psychologically prepared for the procedure, and that all documentation, including laboratory results and reports, are available to the cath lab staff (8).

PRE-PROCEDURE CARE PLAN FOR PATIENTS UNDERGOING AN ELECTROPHYSIOLOGY STUDY/RADIO-FREQUENCY ABLATION

Action	Rationale
Obtain a brief history and check that biographical details and next of kin are correct	Checking the patient's biographical details and next of kin ensures that medical records are up-to-date and that, in the event of an emergency, the correct person is contacted. Record keeping is a fundamental part of nursing care, ensuring high standards of clinical care and improving communication and dissemination of information (19)

Action	Rationale
Explain to the patient and their family what an EPS/ radio-frequency ablation is and what will happen during and after the procedure. Provide an information booklet about the procedure	The period before an invasive procedure may be a time of anxiety and fear, for various reasons. Discussion and reassurance may help to relieve some of these feelings (11)
Check whether the patient is allergic to any food, drugs or other substances. Inform the doctor if the patient is allergic to any potential drugs used in the procedure	Patients with a history of allergy to iodine-containing substances, such as seafood or contrast agents, should be given an antihistamine and steroids before the procedure (30). In addition to this, a non-ionic contrast dye may be used for the procedure (6)
Warfarin should be stopped at least 48 hours prior to the procedure	Warfarin should be withheld for at least 48 hours prior to the procedure, to ensure an international normalised ratio (INR) of less than 2. Patients at high risk for thromboembolism should be admitted for heparinisation while the effects of oral anticoagulation wane (6)
Ideally, INR should be less than 2 (inform the cardiologist if it is higher)	Warfarin interferes with blood coagulation by blocking the effect of vitamin K. It has a long-acting half-life of 36–42 hours. The anticoagulation effect is described in a measurement of the INR. Therefore, any INR measurement of more than 2 increases the patient's risk of bleeding uncontrollably during and/or after the procedure (3)
Ensure that all antiarrhythmic drugs have been stopped for at least five half-lives of the relevant drugs	This is in order to study the arrhythmias without the influence of any drugs (29)
Obtain baseline observations of temperature, pulse and blood pressure and blood glucose. Record a standard 12-lead ECG	In order to provide a baseline, for comparison after the EPS/radio-frequency ablation (30)

Action	Rationale
Check for patent left and right pedal pulse	This information will be used for comparison in evaluating peripheral pulses after the catheterisation procedure (30)
If it is not against the patient's religious beliefs, ensure that the patient has shaved both groins appropriately	Body hair is removed in order to reduce infection risk during catheterisation (14; 30)
Ensure that the patient has a patent intravenous catheter (e.g. venflon)	For the administration of intravenous fluids and drugs administered during the study (1)
Record the patient's height and weight	The amount of some of the drugs prescribed during the procedure may be calculated on the patient's weight (1; 15)
The patient should fast for at least 4–6 hours prior to the EPS/radio-frequency ablation	This is due to the patient's possibly requiring sedation and cardioversion to terminate an induced arrhythmia (1)
Patients may wear dentures, glasses and hearing aids during the procedure	Patients are better able to communicate when dentures and hearing aids are in place. Glasses allow the patient to view the procedure better and help to keep the patient oriented to the surroundings (14; 30). These items can be removed by the lab staff if sedation and cardioversion are required
Ensure that identification and allergy bands are correct, legible and secure	To ensure correct identification and prevent possible problems (30)
Allow patients to empty their bladder before the procedure	To help make them more comfortable (30)
Ensure that consent is obtained by the doctor performing the procedure	Consent for any procedure must be obtained by the doctor performing the procedure and a patient signature obtained. A full explanation of the procedure should be given, outlining the benefits and risks (18)

POST-PROCEDURE CARE PLAN

Goal/aim of care

The nursing care of patients following EPS/radio-frequency ablation is directed towards the prevention and detection of complications.

Action	Rationale
On warding, attach the patient to a cardiac monitor and check pulse and blood pressure	In order to observe the patient's vital signs post procedure (17)
The pulse	Tachycardia (100–120 beats per minute) is not unusual after catheterisation. This may be a sign of anxiety, an indication of fluid loss due to diuresis or a reaction to medication used during the procedure, such as atropine. Fluids, time and reassurance often bring the heart rate down to more normal levels. Heart rates above 120 beats per minute should be evaluated for other causes, such as haemorrhage, more severe fluid imbalance, fever or arrhythmias (30). If not on betablockers, a bradycardia may indicate a vasovagal response. arrhythmias or an infarction and should be assessed by an ECG and correlated with other clinical signs such as pain and blood pressure (30).
Blood pressure	Patients may return to the ward with a low blood pressure caused by drugs, such as vasodilators, administered during the procedure. In addition, the contrast dye acts as an osmotic diuretic and patients may become hypotensive due to volume depletion. Patients are thus kept on bed rest until fluid balance is restored, with oral liquids or by intravenous replacement. If the blood pressure is less than 75–80% of baseline, other causes such as blood loss or arrhythmias must be considered and assessed, and the doctor notified (30)

Action	Rationale
If anaesthetic was administered, monitor the pulse oximetry	Hypoxia occurs for a variety of reasons following anaesthesia. The administration of supplemental oxygen in the immediate post-operative phase will help to reduce the risk of hypoxia occurring. The aim is to maintain normal levels of arterial blood gases and peripheral oxygen saturations (23)
If anaesthetic was administered, monitor the respiratory rate	Anaesthesia and opiates may depress respiration. Although the anaesthetist aims to have reversed these effects by the time the patient is warded, there is potential for severe respiratory depression to be present in the immediate post-procedure period (23)
Pedal pulse	The most frequent complication of percutaneous catheterisation procedures is arterial thrombosis. The puncture site in the groin should be checked for visible bleeding, swelling or tenderness. The arterial pulse at the site and at points distal to it should be compared with pulses on the opposite limb and those recorded before the procedure. Capillary filling and the warmth of the limb should also be evaluated. Blanching, cramping, coolness, pain, numbness or tingling may indicate reduced perfusion and must be carefully evaluated. A diminished or absent pulse is a sign of serious arterial occlusion (14; 30). If a compression device is being used to achieve haemostasis, the pressure should be reduced. If this does not improve circulation, medical staff should be informed (30)
Bleeding and/or haematoma	Research shows that the majority of bleeding/haematoma was detected by nurses checking the groin (5)

Action	Rationale
Until the patient is mobile, check these observations half-hourly and ask the patient to report any feelings of wetness, stickiness, warmth or bleeding in the puncture-site area	Research shows that a large proportion of puncture-site bleeding was detected through the patient's calling for assistance (5)
Advise the patient to keep the affected leg straight whilst on bed rest	Bleeding and haematoma formation may occur when a patient moves the limb too vigorously (14; 30)
If the patient is a diabetic, check their blood sugar on warding	To ensure that the patient is not hypoglycaemic, as they may have fasted for long periods prior to the procedure (30)
Advise patients to inform the nurse if they experience any chest pain	Chest pain may indicate potential cardiac complications; therefore, nurses should be aware of it if it is present (17)
Ensure that any intravenous fluids are running at the correct rate, and administer any drugs prescribed post procedure	It is the ward nurses' responsibility to ensure that the prescribed drugs, intravenous or oral, are administered correctly (17; 20)
Ensure that a post-procedure ECG has been completed	The pre and post ECGs may be used for comparison if the patient develops any chest pain or arrhythmias (14; 17)
If the patient was anaesthetised, ensure that the patient is fully awake before providing them with something to eat or drink	During anaesthesia, voluntary muscular control is temporarily lost; therefore, post procedure, if the patient is not fully awake, fluids may be inhaled accidentally (23). Initially, try patients with sips of water
Once awake, encourage the patient to drink and provide them with something to eat	Patients are often tired, hungry and uncomfortable when they return from the laboratory (30). Patients should be encouraged to drink plenty in order to prevent hypotension (2)
If a vascular closure device was used to achieve haemostasis, such as an AngioSeal, please follow the manufacturer's guidelines	These devices have been shown to reduce the time to obtain haemostasis; therefore, the patient can mobilise as per manufacturers' protocols if no

Action	Rationale
about bed rest and mobilising the patient	problems develop (2; 14). However, the patient may have to remain on the cardiac monitor to observe for any recurrent or iatrogenic arrhythmias overnight (14)
If the patient has the femoral sheaths in situ, the cardiologists will advise when the sheaths should be removed	Femoral sheaths are normally removed 3–4 hours after catheterisation procedures that utilised heparin, to allow time for the heparin to dissipate (17; 18)
Once the femoral sheath has been removed and haemostasis has been achieved, the patient must lie flat for 2 hours and then may sit up for 2 hours	Patients are advised to remain on bed rest in order not to disturb the newly formed clot over the puncture site. However, bed-rest post-sheath removal guidelines vary from hospital to hospital (25). Keeling *et al.* (2000) suggest that lying the patient flat for 2 hours and then sitting them up for 2 hours is usually sufficient to ensure haemostasis (13). However, smaller studies since then indicate that it may be safe to reduce bed rest further (25)
Once mobile, observations may cease, unless the patient complains of numbness, pins and needles or a lump in the groin area or the puncture site begins to bleed	Complications such as bleeding or haematomas are normally observed within 10 minutes of ambulation (16)
Whilst on bed rest, advise patients to press on the puncture site if they cough or sneeze	Patients are advised to press on the puncture site while coughing or sneezing in order to prevent the newly formed clot from being disturbed (5)
Advise patients to take things slowly when they first mobilise	A patient may drop their blood pressure by simply standing up abruptly after prolonged bed rest (27)
Prior to discharge, the patient should be instructed about puncture-site care, and informed of any signs and symptoms which	So that patients will be aware of potential complications post discharge and know what to do in the event of these occurring (14)

Action	Rationale
require a doctor's review. A discharge leaflet should be provided	
Any changes in medication should be discussed with the patient	When discharging a patient, it is the nurses' responsibility to inform the patient about the medication that they have been prescribed so that they will take it correctly at home (20)

REFERENCES

1. Attin, M. (2001) 'Electrophysiology studies: A comprehensive review', *Journal of Critical Care*, **10**(4).
2. Baim, D. S. (2006) *Grossman's Cardiac Catheterisation: Angiography and Intervention*, 7th edn, Philadelphia, PA, Lippincott Williams & Wilkins.
3. Blann, A., Landray, M. and Lip, G. (2002) 'An overview of antithrombotic therapy', *British Medical Journal*, **325**: 762–5.
4. Blomstrom-Ludqvist, C. and Scheinman, M. (2003) *ACC/AHA/ESC Guidelines for the Management of Patients with Supraventricular Arrhythmias*, available online at ACC – *www.acc.org*, AHA – *www.americanheart.org* and ESC – *www.escardio.org*.
5. Botti, M., Williamson, B. and Steen, K. (2001) 'Coronary angiography observations: Evidence-based or ritualistic practice?', *Heart & Lung: The Journal of Acute and Critical Care*, **30**(2): 138–45.
6. Braunweld, E., Zipes, D. and Libby, P. (2001) *Heart Disease: A Textbook of Cardiovascular Medicine*, Vol. 1, 6th edn, London, W.B. Saunders Co.
7. Bubien, R., Knotts, S. and Kay, G. (1995) 'Radiofrequency catheter ablation: Concepts and nursing implications', *Cardiovascular Nursing*, **31**(3): 17–23.
8. Carter, L. and Lamerton, M. (1996) 'Understanding balloon mitral valvuloplasty: The Inoue technique', *Intensive and Critical Care Nursing*, **12**: 147–54.
9. DVLA (2006) *For Medical Practitioners: At a Glance Guide to the Current Medical Standards of Fitness to Drive*, February, available online at *www.dvla.gov.uk*.
10. Garren, C. (1998) 'Radio waves fight SVT', *RN*, **61**(7): 27–31.
11. Hughes, S. (2002) 'The effects of pre-operative information', *Nursing Standard*, **16**: 28, 33–7.
12. Julian, D. G., Cowan, J. C. and McLenachan, J. M. (2005) *Cardiology*, 8th edn, Edinburgh, Elsevier Saunders Co. Ltd.
13. Keeling, A., Fisher, C., Haugh K., Powers, E. and Turner, M. (2000) 'Reducing time in bed after percutaneous transluminal coronary angioplasty (TIBS III)', *American Journal of Critical Care*, **9**(3): 185–7.
14. Kern, M. J. (2003) *The Cardiac Catheterisation Handbook*, 4th edn, London, Mosby.
15. Lemone, P. and Burke, K. (2004) *Medical/Surgical Nursing: Critical Thinking in Client Care*, 3rd edn, Upper Saddle River, NJ, Pearson Prentice Hall.
16. Logemann, T., Luetmer, P., Kaliebe, J., Olson, K. and Murdock, D. (1999) 'Two versus six hours of bed rest following left-sided cardiac catheterisation and a meta-analysis of early ambulation trials', *The American Journal of Cardiology*, **84**: 486–8.

17. Morton, P. G., Fontaine, D. K., Hudak, C. M. and Gallo, B. M. (2005) *Critical Care Nursing: A Holistic Approach*, 8th edn, Philadelphia, PA, Lippincott Williams & Wilkins.

18. Norell, M. and Perrins, J. (2003) *Essential Interventional Cardiology*, Philadelphia, PA, W.B. Saunders Co.

19. Nursing Midwifery Council (2002a) *Guidelines for Records and Record Keeping*, London, Nursing and Midwifery Council, April.

20. Nursing Midwifery Council (2002b) *Guidelines for the Administration of Medicines*, London, Nursing and Midwifery Council.

21. Rosendorff, C. (2005) *Essential Cardiology: Principles and Practice*, 2nd edn, Totowa, NJ, Humana Press.

22. Shea, J. B. (2004) 'Cardiovascular medicine: What you should know about catheter ablation', available online at *www.brighamandwomens.org/cvcenter/Patient/catheterablations.asp*.

23. Sheppard, M. and Wright, M. (2000) *Principles and Practice of High Dependency Nursing*, Edinburgh, Bailliere Tindall.

24. Swanton, R. H. (2003) *Cardiology*, 5th edn, Oxford, Blackwell Publishing.

25. Tagney, J. and Lackie, D. (2005) 'Bed-rest post-femoral arterial sheath removal: What is safe practice? A clinical audit', *British Association of Critical Care Nurses, Nursing in Critical Care*, **10**(4): 167–73.

26. Thompson, P. (1997) *Coronary Care Manual*, London, Churchill Livingstone.

27. Topol, E. J. (1999) *Textbook of Interventional Cardiology*, 3rd edn, London, W.B. Saunders Co.

28. Tracy, C., Akhtar, M., DiMarco, J., Packer, D. and Weitz, H. (2000) 'American College of Cardiology/American Heart Association Clinical Competence Statement on Invasive Electrophysiology Studies, Catheter ablation and Cardioversion', *Circulation*, **102**: 2309–20.

29. Van Riper, S. and Van Riper, J. (1997) *Cardiac Diagnostic Tests: A Guide for Nurses*, Philadelphia, PA, W.B. Saunders Co.

30. Woods, S., Froelicher, E. and Motzer, S. (2000) *Cardiac Nursing*, 4th edn, Philadelphia, PA, Lippincott Williams & Wilkins.

9 Cardioversion

WHAT IS CARDIOVERSION?

Cardioversion is the restoration of the normal heart rhythm from an arrhythmia. There are two ways in which this can be accomplished. First, there is chemical cardioversion, which restores the normal rhythm of the heart by antiarrhythmic drugs (1). The second method is electrical cardioversion, which is also known as direct current (DC) cardioversion. This is the use of an electric shock of brief duration and high energy to terminate a tachyarrhythmia (1). The aim is to cause a momentary discharge of all the cardiac cells to allow the primary pacemaker (sinoatrial (SA) node) to recapture the heart rhythm and stop the arrhythmia (13).

Electrical cardioversion appears to be most effective in terminating those tachyarrhythmias caused by re-entry events, such as atrial flutter and atrial fibrillation (AF), atrioventricular (AV) node re-entry reciprocating tachycardias associated with Wolff–Parkinson–White syndrome, and most forms of ventricular tachycardias, ventricular flutter and ventricular fibrillation (VF) (5). When treating life-threatening tachyarrhythmias such as ventricular tachycardia or VF, the use of direct current electricity is usually called defibrillation. However, as described in this chapter, the elective DC cardioversion of tachyarrhythmias such as AF is a more controlled procedure (13).

WHY ELECTIVELY USE DIRECT CURRENT CARDIOVERSION?

In 1962, Lown first described how using electrical shock successfully converted atrial arrhythmias to sinus rhythm (3). As DC cardioversion has been shown to provide haemodynamic and symptomatic benefits, thereby improving the cardiac rate–response, decreasing the amount of time that patients require in hospital and reducing the risks and/or complications of atrial arrhythmias, DC cardioversion is now widely used (4). Although DC cardioversion can convert atrial flutter and atrial tachycardia to sinus rhythm, it is mainly used to convert persistent AF to sinus rhythm (4), which is why AF is examined in this chapter.

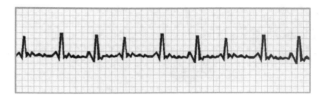

Figure 9.1. ECG strip of atrial fibrillation.

ATRIAL FIBRILLATION

Atrial fibrillation is the most common arrhythmia in clinical practice. The mortality risk of a patient with AF has been reported to be twice as high as somebody with sinus rhythm (3). It is believed that AF stems from the firing of a number of impulses in circuit re-entry pathways in the atria. The atrial impulses occur very fast, and may fire up to 400–600 times per minute, causing the atria to quiver instead of contract (2). This appears as a wavy line on the electrocardiogram (ECG) tracing (Figure 9.1) and is characterised by the absence of *P* waves, with an irregular ventricular response (2).

Atrial fibrillation may cause symptoms such as palpitations, dyspnoea, fatigue, dizziness, chest discomfort, the sensation of being unable to catch one's breath and a decrease in exercise tolerance and well-being (6). These symptoms may be due to a reduction in cardiac output, caused by the rapid ventricular response and the loss of atrial kick (12):

> *Rapid ventricular response*: with the increase in the atrial rate, the ventricular impulses may increase so fast that there is inadequate time for diastolic filling and therefore the cardiac output falls (12).

> *Loss of A–V synchrony/atrial kick*: the amount of blood pumped into the ventricles by the contraction of the atria, which accounts for about 30% of the cardiac output; this is known as 'atrial kick' (2). However, with AF, as the atria are quivering instead of contracting, the atrial kick is lost (2).

Not all patients with AF suffer debilitating symptoms and may survive for many years with few symptoms However, AF is treated as a serious condition, as it increases the patient's risk of developing tachycardiomyopathy (i.e. heart failure) and/or a thrombo-embolic event (i.e. blood clots) (3). Soon after the onset of AF, electrical and mechanical changes occur, referred to as remodelling. These adverse changes, including alterations in how rapidly atrial tissues recover excitability and the enlargement of the atria, are believed to facilitate the development and maintenance of AF, hence the concept 'AF begets AF' (6). This means that the longer somebody is in AF, the harder it will be to convert them to sinus rhythm.

In addition to this, the lack of movement in the quivering atria encourages thrombosis. Therefore, a blood clot (embolism) may form, particularly in patients with mitral valve disease. If an emboli was dislodged from the right atrium, it may produce pulmonary artery obstruction or pulmonary embolism in the lungs, while a dislodged embolism from the left atrium may lodge in cerebral (causing a stroke), renal (causing renal failure) or other peripheral vessels (causing deep vein thrombosis) (12).

CAUSES OF ATRIAL FIBRILLATION

Common causes of AF include:

- rheumatic mitral valve disease;
- ischaemic heart disease, particularly acute myocardial infarction;
- alcohol;
- thyrotoxicosis;
- hypertension;
- acute infections, particularly when these affect the lungs;
- cardiopulmonary surgery;
- a rare complication of many other types of heart disease (12).

Atrial fibrillation may be paroxysmal, with attacks lasting for a few minutes or hours. This is particularly likely in acute myocardial infarction, in chest infections and in the early stages of thyrotoxicosis and mitral valve disease. In rheumatic cases, the arrhythmia usually becomes established eventually and persists for the rest of the patient's life (12). Therefore, AF has been classified into three groups.

CLASSIFICATION OF ATRIAL FIBRILLATION

Atrial fibrillation has been classified into three groups:

- *Paroxysmal*. Self-terminating at least once. Patients may be unaware of bursts of AF.
- *Persistent*. More than 48 hours with no spontaneous termination. Can be converted to sinus rhythm with drugs or DC cardioversion.
- *Permanent*. Established AF. Cannot be terminated by drugs or DC cardioversion. Patients need rate-control therapy plus consideration of anticoagulation (19).

There is a gradual tendency over time for paroxysmal AF to become persistent and, finally, permanent. However, of these three classifications, only persistent AF is suitable for DC cardioversion (19).

   In general, if AF lasts less than 48 hours, antiarrhythmic drugs (AADs) are highly effective and peri-cardioversion anticoagulation treatment is not needed (see 'Anticoagulation', overleaf). On the other hand, if AF duration is more than 48 hours, the likelihood of pharmacological conversion decreases. In these patients, DC cardioversion after adequate anticoagulation treatment is preferred (3).

Electrical cardioversion offers obvious advantages over drug therapy in terminating tachycardia, such as:

- A precisely regulated 'dose' of electricity can restore sinus rhythm immediately and safely.
- The distinction between supraventricular and ventricular tachyarrhythmias – crucial to the proper medical management of arrhythmias – becomes less significant.
- The time-consuming titration of drugs with potential side effects is avoided (5).

ANTICOAGULATION

Patients undergoing pharmacological or electrical cardioversion are at risk of thromboembolism, as, if a clot is present, the resuming of normal atrial contraction may actually dislodge the clot (13). If the left atrium is small and AF has only been present for 24–48 hours prior to cardioversion, anticoagulation is unnecessary. However, if the left atrium is dilated, there is mitral valve disease or AF has been prolonged, then the patient should be anticoagulated with warfarin for 4 weeks prior to DC cardioversion. The risk of systemic emboli is about 5–7% without anticoagulation and less than 1.6% with it. Patients with spontaneous echo contrast in the left atria (thought to be a prelude to thrombi) should also be anticoagulated (19).

Anticoagulation with warfarin for at least 4 weeks after the DC cardioversion is recommended, because restoration of mechanical function lags behind that of electrical systolic function, and thrombi can still form in largely akinetic atria, although they are electrocardiographically in sinus rhythm. Importantly, exclusion of left atrial thrombus by transoesophageal echocardiography may not always preclude embolism after cardioversion of AF (5).

Atrial thrombi may be present in patients with non-fibrillation atrial tachyarrhythmias such as atrial flutter and congenital heart disease. The same pre-cardioversion and post-cardioversion anticoagulation recommendations apply to these patients as well as to those with AF (5).

WHEN SHOULD PATIENTS HAVE DIRECT CURRENT CARDIOVERSION?

The Resuscitation Council United Kingdom (2000) has attempted to simplify the management options for AF by devising a treatment algorithm. The algorithm is divided into three pathways: high, intermediate and low risk. The pathway chosen is dependent on the heart rate and the patient's condition (13):

High risk. A patient is defined as high risk if the heart rate is greater than 150 beats per minute (bpm) and the patient is symptomatic. Treatment with intravenous heparin and electrical cardioversion should be immediate. If this fails, pharmacological cardioversion with intravenous amiodarone of 300 mg should be attempted. A further dose of 300 mg amiodarone can be infused, if required (13).

Intermediate risk. Intermediate risk is defined as a heart rate of between 100 and 150 bpm and is dependent on whether underlying cardiac disease is present, the time of onset of AF and whether the patient is compromised. If no structural heart disease is present, the patient is not compromised and AF duration is greater than 24 hours, then the emphasis is to control the heart rate, using betablockers, calcium antagonists and digoxin. Cardioversion should be attempted after the patient has received 3–4 weeks of anticoagulation. If the duration of AF is less than 24 hours, then the aim is to restore sinus rhythm with intravenous amiodarone/flecainide or DC shock (13).

Low risk. Patients are identified as low risk if they have a heart rate of less than 100 bpm and have no symptoms. If the duration of AF is less than 24 hours, treatment is aimed at restoring sinus rhythm with intravenous heparin and intravenous amiodarone/flecainide or DC shock. If, however, the duration of AF exceeds 24 hours, cardioversion should be planned for 3–4 weeks following anticoagulation (13).

PREPARING A PATIENT FOR A DIRECT CURRENT CARDIOVERSION

As the majority of patients will undergo electrical cardioversion as a planned admission, they may be invited to attend a pre-admission clinic. Attending a pre-admission clinic provides the nursing staff with the opportunity to explain to the patient and their family/carers what cardioversion entails and what they can expect to happen on the day, and allows opportunities to ask questions in order to reduce their anxieties (13). It also provides the opportunity to advise patients to omit any diuretics, digoxin or oral hypoglycaemic medications and/or reduce their insulin appropriately on the day of the cardioversion (4).

In addition to completing the patient's biographical details, allergy status and previous medical history, completing an ECG whilst attending the pre-admission clinic will reveal whether the patient has reverted to sinus rhythm spontaneously and thus does not need the cardioversion (1).

It also provides the opportunity to check the patient's bloods, such as:

INR (an internationally recognised ratio of a patient's blood's ability to clot). It is recommended that patients with AF should have an INR of between 2 and 3 before they are cardioverted (20).

Urea&Electrolytes. As high or low potassium levels may encourage cardiac arrhythmias (20), it is recommended to keep the serum potassium between 4.5 and 5.5 mmol/l, if possible (19).

Serum digoxin. Levels may also indicate how well the patient is digitalised (normal range is 0.8–1.8 mg/ml). Cardioversion in digoxin toxicity can produce dangerous ventricular arrhythmias (1). Because of the dangers of digoxin toxicity, it has become common practice to stop digoxin for 24–48 hours before cardioversion. However, cardioversion in the presence of therapeutic levels of digoxin is safe. There is no need to postpone the cardioversion if the patient is receiving standard doses of digoxin, when the renal function and plasma electrolytes are normal, and there are no symptoms or ECG findings suggestive of digoxin toxicity (1). Therefore, unless digoxin toxicity is suspected, it is not necessary to routinely check serum digoxin levels prior to cardioversion.

During pre-admission clinic, the patient may undergo an echocardiogram to measure their heart and to look for emboli forming. An echocardiogram uses ultrasound to obtain images of the heart. There are two ways to obtain an echocardiogram. The transthoracic echocardiogram is a type of non-invasive ultrasound in which the probe obtains the image of the heart. The probe is placed on the outside of the chest and it is commonly performed to measure left atrial size, left ventricle (LV) dimensions, such as LV wall thickness, LV function and movement, and also to establish whether blood clot formation or valvular heart disease is present. The transoesophageal echocardiogram (TOE) is a more invasive form of ultrasound imaging used to investigate the heart. The patient is starved for 6 hours before the procedure and informed consent should be obtained. The patient is given mild sedation and a local-anaesthetic spray is applied to the back of the throat to block the gag reflex. A flexible endoscopic probe is passed via the mouth and positioned in the oesophagus directly behind the heart (19). This provides superior-quality cardiac images and is especially useful to identify thrombi and is, therefore, often used as a guide to cardioversion risk (12). The patient remains nil-by-mouth until the gag reflex returns (13).

If the patient does not attend pre-admission clinic, a TOE may be used immediately before cardioversion to help exclude atrial clotting (13). Recent experience with TOE has shown that thrombi in the atrial appendage occur in about 13% of patients with AF. If no thrombi are seen on TOE, then DC cardioversion may be performed safely without prior anticoagulation; however, if a TOE is not available, then patients should be anticoagulated beforehand (19).

CONSIDERATIONS USING DIFFERENT PADDLES

Traditionally, the shock is delivered with two electrode paddles (1) (Figure 9.2(a)). However, self-adhesive pads have proved to have transthoracic impedance similar to paddles and are very useful in elective cardioversions (5) (Figure 9.2(b)). When using paddles, electrode jelly may be applied to the skin under the paddles in order to achieve good electrical contact and to avoid burning the skin. However, it is essential to avoid spreading jelly between the two paddles. Alternatively, pads impregnated with electrode gel may be used. These prevent jelly being spread over inappropriate areas, including the operator (1).

Correct positioning is essential. Usually, one electrode is placed at the level of the cardiac apex, close to the midaxillary line, and the other is positioned to the

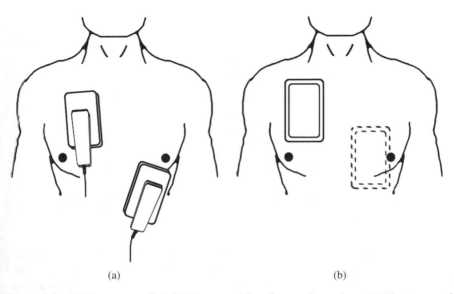

(a)   (b)

Figure 9.2. (a) Placement of defibrillator paddles for cardioversion. (b) Placement of defibrillator self-adhesive pads for cardioversion.

right of the upper sternum. Alternatively, a flat paddle, or self-adhesive pad, can be placed beneath the patient's back, behind the heart, and a second paddle positioned over the precordium. Standard paddles can be applied anteroposteriorly if the patient is turned onto his or her side – one paddle is placed over the precordium and the other paddle below the left shoulder to the left of the spine (1).

Research has not identified one electrode position's being superior to another and current guidelines reflect this (13). Thus, positioning of the electrodes is at the operator's discretion. However, if a patient has a pacemaker, consideration should be given to lead positioning, as cardioversion may cause pacemaker damage unless the paddles are at least 15 cm from the generator and preferably are positioned so that they are at right angles to the line between the pacemaker generator and the heart. Pacemaker function should be checked after the procedure (1).

INTERNAL DIRECT CURRENT CARDIOVERSION

In 2–5% of patients with AF, sinus rhythm cannot be restored by external shocks, despite all the above measures, including ibutilide pretreatment. Very obese patients or those with severe obstructive lung disease are most frequently affected. In such cases, internal cardioversion can be performed by using standard percutaneous access to introduce specially configured catheters into the atria to deliver a shock. Internal shocks ranging from 2–15 joules are able to terminate AF in more than 90% of patients whose arrhythmia did not terminate with transthoracic shocks (5).

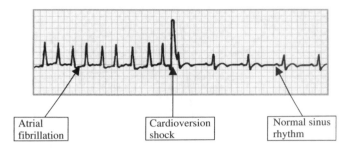

Figure 9.3. ECG strip showing cardioversion shock.

SYNCHRONISATION IN ELECTIVE DIRECT CURRENT CARDIOVERSION

Cardioversion is carried out in a similar way to defibrillation, except that cardioversion is more controlled – a synchronised rather than an asynchronous shock (as in VF) is administered (13). Ventricular fibrillation may be induced if a shock coincides with the ventricular T wave; therefore, defibrillators have a mechanism whereby discharge is triggered to occur on the R or S wave. This mechanism should be used during cardioversion for all arrhythmias except VF. With VF, there will be no detectable R wave and, thus, if the mechanism is in operation, the defibrillator will not discharge (1) (Figure 9.3).

ENERGY REQUIRED FOR DIRECT CURRENT CARDIOVERSION

The amount of shock energy required depends on the rhythm being converted and whether a monophasic or biphasic defibrillator is being used. Biphasic shocks deliver electrical current in a positive direction for a specified time; the current is then reversed to flow in a negative direction for the remainder of the discharge. This technology offers the same or better chance of success and uses less energy than monophasic shocks, which send the current in a single direction between electrodes (13).

Although recommendations are made for the number of joules needed to convert various rhythms, the actual energy needed varies with the duration of the dysrhythmia, rate, morphology and the underlying cause of the dysrhythmias, as well as transthoracic impedance (17). In general, low energy levels are used initially. If unsuccessful, further shocks can be given at increased levels (1). The amount of shock energy recommended for monophasic cardioversion of AF is to give 100 joules to start, followed by 200 joules if the patient remains in AF, and then 360 joules or the biphasic equivalent. It may be appropriate to select lower energies of 50–100 joules if the duration of AF is less than 24 hours, the patient has no structural heart disease and antiarrhythmic drugs are not being administered (13). Supraventricular arrhythmias, namely atrial flutter and supraventricular tachycardia, usually respond to low-energy shocks; 50 joules is a suitable initial level (1).

WHAT A PATIENT CAN EXPECT WHEN UNDERGOING A DC CARDIOVERSION

PRIOR TO THE PROCEDURE

After checking that the patient's biographical details have been completed appropriately, another ECG should be completed to ensure that the patient has not reverted to sinus rhythm spontaneously (1).

When the patient is provided with a gown, they should be recommended to wear it with the ties facing the front in order to make it easier to apply the paddles. The patient will be attached to a heart monitor or ECG in order to monitor their heart rhythm throughout the procedure.

Because the procedure is painful, electrical cardioversion needs to be performed under anaesthetic. However, some centres perform electrical cardioversion under sedation, using diazepam or midazolam, which has been shown to be safe and effective (13). Therefore, prior to the procedure, the patient will be assessed by an anaesthetist, who will take a detailed history, looking at issues such as past medical history, chronic illness, reaction to previous anaesthetics and current state of health (18). A combination of inhalational and intravenous anaesthetic may be used. Intravenous agents produce a rapid induction for the patient, which is more pleasant than breathing through a mask, whilst inhalational agents provide maintenance of anaesthesia. Although the inhalational agents are excreted through the lungs, allowing rapid emergence from unconsciousness, the intravenous agents need to be metabolised and excreted by the body, so patients may be drowsy when returning to the ward (18). The anaesthetist may prescribe a pre-medication to reduce anxiety and produce some sedation (10). These should be administered 45–70 minutes prior to the procedure, but only after the consent form has been signed, as they can make a patient drowsy (10).

DURING THE PROCEDURE

Once the patient has been sedated/anaesthetised, the steps for cardioversion are as follows:

1. Turn on the defibrillator and monitor, and attach the monitoring electrodes to the patient's chest. Avoid placing the electrodes in the area where the defibrillator paddles/pads will be positioned. Some devices perform both monitoring and defibrillation through disposable defibrillation patches.

2. Select a monitoring lead that provides a good ECG pattern with a tall *R* wave. If monitoring is by way of the disposable defibrillator patches, select the 'paddles' lead.
3. Turn on the synchroniser mode button. The size of the *R* wave on the monitored lead may need to be adjusted until the synchronisation marker appears on each *R* wave.
4. Sedate the patient, and maintain adequate airway.
5. Either remove the paddles from the defibrillator and apply generous amounts of gel to them, and then firmly place them against the chest wall. Care should be taken not to smear electrode gel between the between the two paddles on the chest.
6. Alternatively, gel pads or pre-gelled defibrillator patches can be placed in the appropriate positions on the chest wall. This is done to prevent skin burns and decrease electrical resistance. When using patches, be sure that there are no air pockets by applying the patches firmly from the centre to the periphery. Air pockets can cause skin burns.
7. Apply paddles/patches, one just below the right clavicle and the other over the apex of the heart. If the anterior–posterior patches are used, place the posterior one behind the heart in the left infra-scapular location. Make sure that the paddles/patches are away from an implanted pacemaker or implantable cardioverter–defibrillator generator.
8. Set the desired energy level.
9. Press the charge button. A light will flash until the paddles are fully charged.
10. Reconfirm the synchronisation markers on the *R* waves on the monitor.
11. Call out 'clear' to make sure nobody is touching the patient or the bed.
12. Discharge the paddle while applying firm pressure. Push and hold both paddles' discharge buttons until the defibrillator discharges. Maintain contact on the chest wall until the machine has delivered the shock. There will be a momentary delay from the pressing on the discharge button to delivery of the shock because of the synchronisation with the *R* wave. Failure to keep paddles on the chest wall can result in failure of the cardioversion and burns to the chest.
13. Remove the paddles and observe the patient's vital signs.
14. Subsequent shocks may need to be delivered. If so, be certain to select the synchronisation mode.
15. If the patient's rhythm deteriorates to VF, turn off the synchroniser and immediately defibrillate the patient, starting with 200 joules and increasing to 360 joules, as needed.
16. Once the patient is in sinus rhythm, return them to the ward for observation (17).

POST PROCEDURE

On warding, the patient is attached to a cardiac monitor to observe for cardiac arrhythmias which are common in the early stages post-cardioversion, the most common being bradycardia and heart block (13). Post-shock arrhythmias usually are transient and do not require therapy (5). Ventricular arrhythmias are less common and are usually the result of poor operator technique or digoxin toxicity (13).

Once the patient has recovered from the anaesthetic and is able to mobilise, the cardiac monitoring may be discontinued.

DISCHARGE ADVICE

Patients are normally discharged on the day of the cardioversion, once they have recovered from the anaesthetic. This can be identified when there is a return of O_2 to baseline; stable vital signs; a return of level of consciousness to baseline; and a return of baseline ambulation capability (4).

When discharging patients, it is good practice to provide written instruction advising patients:

1. not to drive or operate complex appliances or machinery for 24 hours;
2. to resume diet, but no alcohol for 24 hours;
3. to resume medication with or without changes;
4. to make a follow-up appointment;
5. to arrange to have their INR checked (4).

COMPLICATIONS

Apart from slight skin burns, the procedure is usually free from undesirable effects (12). Transient arrhythmias occasionally occur but these are rarely a problem unless there is digoxin toxicity (1). Embolic episodes are reported to occur in 1–3% of the patients converted from AF to sinus rhythm (5).

CARE PLANS

PROBLEM/NEED

Patient is to have an elective electrical cardioversion.

NURSING CONSIDERATION BEFORE THE PROCEDURE

Goal/aim of care

The primary aim of nursing care prior to cardioversion is to maximise patient safety and comfort during the procedure and optimise conditions for a successful outcome. This is achieved by ensuring that the patient is physically and psychologically prepared for the procedure, and that all documentation, including laboratory results and reports, are available to the cath lab staff (7).

PRE-PROCEDURE CARE PLAN FOR PATIENTS UNDERGOING
A CARDIOVERSION

Action	Rationale
Obtain a brief history and check that biographical details and next of kin are correct	Checking the patient's biographical details and next of kin ensures that medical records are up-to-date and, in the event of an emergency, the correct person is contacted. Record keeping is a fundamental part of nursing care, ensuring high standards of clinical care and improving communication and dissemination of information (15)
Explain the procedure to the patient and significant others to alleviate anxieties	The period before any procedure may cause extreme anxiety in some patients. Discussion and reassurance may help to relieve some of these feelings (9)
Check to see whether the patient has stopped their digoxin	Ideally, digoxin would be stopped 36 hours prior to electrical cardioversion, as it can be pro-arrhythmic, and may affect a positive outcome, namely the patient does not convert to sinus rhythm (1)
Record an ECG	An ECG should be obtained to ensure that the patient is still in AF/flutter/tachycardia. Other non-life-threatening arrhythmias are not amenable to cardioversion (1)
Cannulate the patient	To provide intravenous access to administer prescribed drugs (21)
Obtain blood samples for:	
urea and electrolytes	To ensure that sodium and potassium levels are within normal limits. Too low or too high levels may precipitate VF or tachycardia post shock (20). Patients with renal inefficiency are unsuitable for some anaesthetic agents

Action	Rationale
full blood count	To check for any signs of infection, namely raised white cell count; an anaesthetist may be unwilling to anaesthetise a patient with infection, particularly chest infection. A haemoglobin level is obtained to detect for anaemia; again, an anaesthetist may be unwilling to anaesthetise, as this may result in post-anaesthesia complications (8)
INR (aim for levels between 2 and 3)	This result must be between 2 and 3 to reduce the risk of thrombo-embolic events post cardioversion. Anticoagulation should commence at least 4 weeks prior to the procedure (13). Patients in AF are at increased risk of clots forming in the left atrium due to ineffective emptying. A part of this clot may dislodge, resulting in systemic emboli, causing disability or death (13)
Record the patient's height and weight	Height and weight are recorded so that the anaesthetist can ascertain the correct dosage of drugs to administer (10)
Obtain baseline observations of pulse, blood pressure, temperature and blood glucose	This information should be evaluated to ensure that the patient is suitable for the procedure (5). In order to provide a baseline, for comparison after the cardioversion (21)
The patient should fast for at least 4–6 hours prior to the procedure	Patients should be instructed to have no food intake 4 hours prior to admission and no fluids 2 hours prior to admission to avoid the risk of aspiration during anaesthesia (1)

Action	Rationale
Remove dentures, artificial eyes, contact lenses and prosthetics	These items may cause confusion when the anaesthetist is assessing the unconscious patient (14)
Ensure that identification and allergy bands are correct, legible and secure	To ensure correct identification and prevent possible problems (21)
Allow patients to empty their bladder before the procedure	To help make them more comfortable (21)
Ensure that consent is obtained by the doctor performing the procedure	Consent for any procedure must be obtained by the doctor performing the procedure and a patient signature obtained. A full explanation of the procedure should be given, outlining the benefits and risks (14)

POST PROCEDURE

The nursing care of patients following DC cardioversion is directed towards the prevention and detection of complications.

Action	Rationale
On warding, attach the patient to a cardiac monitor and check the heart rate, blood pressure, pulse oximetry and respiratory rate	In order to observe the patient's vital signs post procedure (17)
Heart rate	To observe for cardiac arrhythmias which are common in the early stages post cardioversion, the most common being bradycardia and heart block (13)
Blood pressure	Anaesthetic agents affect blood pressure in various ways, and may cause hypotension (17)
Pulse oximetry	Hypoxia occurs for a variety of reasons following anaesthesia. The administration of supplemental oxygen in the immediate post-operative phase will help to reduce the risk of hypoxia occurring. The aim is to maintain

Action	Rationale
	normal levels of arterial blood gases and peripheral oxygen saturations (18)
Respiratory rate	Anaesthesia and opiates may depress respiration. Although the anaesthetist aims to have reversed these effects by the time the patient is warded, there is potential for severe respiratory depression to be present in the immediate post-procedure period (18)
If the patient is a diabetic, check their blood sugar on warding	To ensure that the patient is not hypoglycaemic, as they may have fasted for long periods prior to the procedure (21)
Inspect the chest wall for signs of burns and treat appropriately	To make the patient more comfortable (17)
Ensure that the patient is fully awake before providing them with something to eat or drink	During anaesthesia, voluntary muscular control is temporarily lost; therefore, post procedure, if the patient is not fully awake, fluids may be inhaled accidentally (18). Initially, try patients with sips of water
The patient should remain on bed rest until all the effects of the anaesthetic have worn off	The patient should remain in bed until effects of the anaesthetic have worn off to prevent accidents such as falls (13)
Any changes in medication should be discussed with the patient	When discharging a patient, it is the nurses' responsibility to inform the patient about the medication that they have been prescribed so that they will take it correctly at home (16)
If the patient has a pacemaker/ICD implant, these should be checked after DC cardioversion	The pacemaker may need to be reprogrammed, as a temporary rise in capture thresholds may follow DC cardioversion. Older pacemaker models may revert to a re-set or back-up mode (17)

Action	Rationale
The patient should be seen by a doctor prior to discharge	The patient should be seen by a doctor prior to discharge and any change in medication and follow-up appointments should be discussed. Recurrence of AF is common, although antiarrhythmic drug therapy often effectively decreases the frequency as measured by time to first recurrence and the arrhythmia-free period (5)

REFERENCES

1. Bennett, D. H. (2002) *Cardiac Arrhythmias: Practical Notes on Interpretation and Treatment*, London, Arnold.
2. Beverage, D., Haworth, K., Labus, D., Mayer, B. and Munson, S. (2005) *ECG Interpretation Made Incredibly Easy*, London, Lippincott Williams & Wilkins.
3. Blaauw, Y., Van Gelder, I. C., Crijns, H. J. G. M. (2002) 'Treatment of atrial fibrillation', *Heart*, **88**(4): 432–7.
4. Botkin, S. B., Dhanekula, L. S. and Olshansky, B. (2003) 'Outpatient cardioversion of atrial arrhythmias: Efficacy, safety, and costs', *American Heart Journal*, **145**(2): 233–8.
5. Braunwald, E., Zipes, D. and Libby, P. (2001) *Heart Disease: A Textbook of Cardiovascular Medicine*, 6th edn, Philadelphia, PA, W.B. Saunders Co.
6. Bubien, R. and Sanchez, J. (2001) 'Atrial fibrillation: Treatment rationale and clinical utility of nonpharmacologic therapies', *AACN Clinical Issues: Advanced Practice in Acute & Critical Care*, **12**(1): 140–55.
7. Carter, L. and Lamerton, M. (1996) 'Understanding balloon mitral valvuloplasty: The Inoue technique', *Intensive and Critical Care Nursing*, **12**: 147–54.
8. Hand, H. (2001) 'Blood and the classification of anaemia', *Nursing Standard*, **15**(39): 45–53.
9. Hughes, S. (2002) 'The effects of pre-operative information', *Nursing Standard*, **16**(28): 33–7.
10. Lemone, P. and Burke, K. (2004) *Medical/Surgical Nursing: Critical Thinking in Client Care*, 3rd edn, Upper Saddle River, NJ, Pearson Prentice Hall.
11. Lown, B. (1962) 'Electrical reversion of cardiac arrhythmias', *British Heart Journal*, **29**: 469–89.
12. Julian, D. G., Cowan, J. C. and McLenachan, J. M. (2005) *Cardiology*, 8th edn, Edinburgh, Elsevier Saunders Co. Ltd.
13. Navas, S. (2003) 'Atrial fibrillation: Part 2', *Nursing Standard*, **17**(38): 47–56.
14. Norell, M. and Perrins, J. (2003) *Essential Interventional Cardiology*, Philadelphia, PA, W.B. Saunders Co.
15. Nursing Midwifery Council (2002a) *Guidelines for Records and Record Keeping*, London, Nursing and Midwifery Council, April.
16. Nursing Midwifery Council (2002b) *Guidelines for the Administration of Medicines*, London, Nursing and Midwifery Council.

17. Morton, P. G., Fontaine, D. K., Hudak, C. M. and Gallo, B. M. (2005) *Critical Care Nursing: A Holistic Approach*, 8th edn, Philadelphia, PA, Lippincott Williams & Wilkins.
18. Sheppard, M. and Wright, M. (2000) *Principles and Practice of High Dependency Nursing*, Edinburgh, Bailliere Tindall.
19. Swanton, R. (2003) *Cardiology*, 5th edn, Oxford, Blackwell Science.
20. Task Force Report (2001) 'ACC/AHA/ESC guidelines for the management of patients with atrial fibrillation', *European Heart Journal*, **22**(20): 1852–923.
21. Woods, S., Froelicher, E. and Motzer, S. (2000) *Cardiac Nursing*, 4th edn, Philadelphia, PA, Lippincott Williams & Wilkins.

10   Temporary Pacemakers

WHAT IS TEMPORARY PACING?

A pacemaker is defined as a battery-operated pulse generator that initiates and controls the electrical stimulation of the heart via one or more electrodes that are in direct contact with the myocardium (4). When a patient requires a pacemaker for a short period of time, the pulse generator will be kept outside the body; this is known as a temporary pacemaker (7). Several types of temporary pacemakers are available, including transvenous, epicardial, transthoracic and transcutaneous (3).

INDICATIONS FOR A TEMPORARY PACEMAKER

Temporary pacing is used in both emergency and elective situations (8). It is indicated in any patient with profound bradycardia and haemodynamic compromise (1). The patient may show signs of decreased cardiac output, such as hypotension or syncope. The temporary pacemaker supports the patient until the condition resolves or until a permanent pacemaker is inserted (3).

Emergencies which compromise a patient's haemodynamic status, thus potentially requiring a temporary pacemaker, include:

- Cardiac arrest followed by *P*-wave asystole (8).
- New-onset second/third AV block in which the patient is symptomatic and not responding to drugs, until a permanent pacemaker can be inserted (14).
- Heart block following myocardial infarction (MI) – the need for pacing after acute MI is related to the site of the MI, its extent and the type of block it may cause (1). The AV node and the bundle branches may be damaged or irritated during an MI, causing heart block. This is usually benign and temporary, so the patient will only need a temporary pacemaker if they develop a symptomatic bradycardia (14).
- Drug-induced symptomatic bradycardia – antiarrhythmic drugs, such as betablockers, calcium channel blockers, digoxin, reserpine and parasympathomimetic agents, can lead to bradycardia, more so in patients with idiosyncratic reactions and conduction system disease. With these drugs, bradycardia may occur even at low blood levels. Therefore, temporary pacing may be required until the drug's action or effects have dissipated. If the

patient needs to be on these drugs for the long term, such as treating ventricular arrhythmias with antiarrhythmic drugs, the patient may need to have a permanent pacemaker inserted (10).

- Pace-terminating rapid supraventricular tachyarrhythmias – the pacemaker paces the heart at a rate faster than its intrinsic rate to override the source of the tachyarrhythmia. When the pacing stimulation ceases, the tachyarrhythmia should break (3). For example, the atria is paced at rapid rates of 200–500 impulses per minute in an attempt to terminate atrial tachyarrhythmias such as atrial tachycardias, atrial flutter and atrial fibrillation. This type of pacing is most frequently performed post cardiac surgery using temporary epicardial leads. It can also be performed using a transvenous lead in the atrium but this method is less effective (14).

Temporary pacemakers may be electively inserted as a prophylactic measure to prevent haemodynamic compromise during the following procedures:

- To provide cover during the cardioversion of supraventricular arrhythmias for patients with bradycardia–tachycardia syndrome (2).
- Patients with pre-existing left bundle branch block are at increased risk of developing complete heart block during right-heart catheterisation (Chapter 4), where the catheter contacts the right bundle branch (1).
- Before surgery, anaesthesia can increase pre-existing block. Patients with asymptomatic heart block should be assessed for a temporary pacemaker prior to any surgery, as vagal influences may produce prolonged sinus arrest (11).
- Temporary epicardial pacing is used after cardiac surgery if the patient develops arrhythmias, or if cardiac output needs to be temporarily augmented. It can also be used to provide atrial overdrive pacing, in an attempt to terminate atrial fibrillation or atrial flutter after cardiac surgery (14).

Temporary pacing wires are usually removed within 72 hours after the resumption of sinus rhythm, but can be left in situ for up to 2 weeks. However, the risk of secondary infection increases the longer the temporary pacemaker is inserted (4). Prolonged use of a temporary pacemaker also increases the risk of lead dislodgement and cardiac perforation (1). Therefore, should persistent conduction defects occur, a permanent device would need to be inserted (4).

TYPES OF TEMPORARY PACEMAKER

TRANSCUTANEOUS PACING

Transcutaneous pacing is a non-invasive method of temporarily pacing the heart in an emergency. It provides safe and effective temporary pacing support for patients in brady-asystolic cardiac arrest (4). One large electrode is placed on the patient's anterior chest wall and a second is applied to his/her back (3).

An electric current is passed through the chest from these electrodes and the voltage is gradually increased until it is of sufficient magnitude to pace the heart. Unfortunately, this is inevitably accompanied by extensive skeletal muscle contractions, which are extremely uncomfortable for the patient (7). Therefore, transcutaneous pacing is normally only used in an emergency, until a transvenous pacemaker can be inserted (3). The patient may need to be sedated if they are alert when a transcutaneous pacemaker is being used (8).

TRANSTHORACIC PACING

Transthoracic pacing is a temporary pacing method used as a last resort in an emergency situation. This method involves inserting a pacing electrode into the right ventricle's myocardium by inserting a needle through the chest wall. Transthoracic pacing has a limited success rate and a high potential for complications such as pericardial tamponade (8). Therefore, it is only used in cases of cardiac arrest, in which asystole is present with P waves (4).

EPICARDIAL PACING

Epicardial pacemakers are commonly used for patients undergoing cardiac surgery. The doctor attaches the tips of the lead wires to the outside surface of the heart and brings the wires out through the chest wall, below the incision. They are then attached to the pulse generator. The lead wires are usually removed several days after surgery or when the patient no longer requires them (3).

TRANSVENOUS PACING

The transvenous pacemaker is probably the most common and reliable type of temporary pacemaker. It is usually inserted at the bedside or in a fluoroscopy suite (3). The pacing electrodes are introduced under local anaesthesia into a systemic vein and advanced with the aid of x-ray screening into the right ventricle or atrium and then connected to the pulse generator (2).

Five different veins may be used, depending on the doctor's preference, pre-existing conditions, or both. Each approach has its advantages and drawbacks. Consideration must also be given to the probability of permanent pacing because the vein cannot be reused once a cut-down procedure has been performed. Veins which can be used are the subclavian, external jugular or internal jugular, antecubital vein and femoral vein (14).

SUBCLAVIAN VEIN, EXTERNAL JUGULAR OR INTERNAL JUGULAR PUNCTURE

The use of the Seldinger technique has almost eliminated the need for a cut-down procedure; subsequently, the neck and shoulder veins have become common sites to insert the transvenous wires (13). In the intensive care unit, the internal jugular and subclavian veins are preferred, because it is easier to insert a pacing wire, provides more stability and has a longer dwell time with less risk of thrombosis or infection (1). In addition, the patient is able to ambulate freely without risk of lead dislodgement (13). Although rare in experienced hands, possible complications include pneumothorax, haemothorax, subclavian artery puncture and air embolism (2).

Unlike the femoral or antecubital veins, these veins do not need fluoroscopy for the placement of a pacing catheter. Instead, a balloon-tipped catheter pacing lead can be floated into place using the internal jugular or subclavian vein as access (1).

ANTECUBITAL VEIN CUT-DOWN

Another option is using one of the antecubital veins, particularly the basilic vein, which takes a more direct course to the central vasculature than the cephalic vein. Antecubital access reduces the risk of bleeding in patients who are anticoagulated or have received thrombolytic therapy, but the patient must keep the arm nearly immobile to minimise the risk of perforation or dislodgement (1). Arm motion can cause a high incidence of electrode movement and displacement, which can stop the pacing or perforate the ventricle. This disadvantage means that the patient will be unable to flex the arm and therefore unable to eat and wash without assistance (13). In addition, poor electrode stability, infection and phlebitis are common complications of this site (2).

FEMORAL VEIN PUNCTURE

The femoral site is frequently used when a temporary pacemaker is inserted prophylactically in the electrophysiology laboratory or catheterisation laboratory, since the need for the temporary pacemaker is usually short-term, sterile technique is easily observed, the patient remains essentially immobile and fluoroscopy is readily available (1).

This method is very easy and quick, provided that the pulse in the femoral artery adjacent to the vein is easy to palpate. However, it should be reserved for short-term emergency purposes because electrode stability is poor and there is a risk of venous thrombosis (2). If phlebitis does occur, it is of a more serious nature in the femoral area because of major vein involvement (13).

Some patients with femoral catheters are allowed to ambulate. If walking is limited, the incidence of complications is low. There are many psychological benefits to the patient who is permitted to be out of bed. When assisting the patient to get up and sit in the chair, care should be taken that hip flexion is minimal (13).

WHAT THE PATIENT MAY EXPECT DURING THE LEAD PLACEMENT

Insertion of a temporary pacing catheter may be performed in a cardiac catheterisation laboratory or at the bedside (with or without the use of fluoroscopy) (14).

Temporary cardiac pacing is most frequently undertaken using the Seldinger technique via the subclavian or jugular vein (7). Therefore, it will be this procedure only that is described in this chapter.

If the temporary pacemaker is being inserted on the ward as an emergency, ensure that the resuscitation trolley is easily accessible and that venous access is available to give drugs if necessary. Brady or tachyarrhythmias are often induced during the procedure, so ensure that atropine, isoprenaline, adrenaline and lignocaine are readily at hand should they be needed. As external transcutaneous pacing can provide short-term support until the temporary pacing wire is inserted, this should be available as well (9).

If time permits, the procedure should be explained to the patient and their family. The teaching should be geared to their level of understanding. Often, although the physician has talked with the patient, the procedure may need to be explained in simpler terms by the nurse (13).

In order to find the subclavian vein, the patient should be advised that they may be positioned lying flat or, if possible, in a slightly head-down position. Alternatively, their legs may be raised to aid venous return and hence distension of the subclavian vein (2). Then their skin is anaesthetised about 1 cm below the mid-point of the clavicle, using a local anaesthetic (7).

When fully numb, following strict surgical asepsis, using the Seldinger technique, a sheath with a non-return valve will be placed in the subclavian/jugular vein, to allow easy manipulation of the wire (9). The pacing wire is passed to the right atrium under fluoroscopic control and rotated until it points downwards and to the patient's left. Then, it is threaded through the tricuspid valve into the left ventricle. The patient should be warned that when the pacing wire is advanced across the tricuspid valve, they may develop an arrhythmia which they might be able to feel. They should be reassured that these arrhythmias usually settle rapidly and require no treatment (9). The wire should be positioned along the floor of the ventricle with its tip in the apex (7). If a dual-chamber temporary pacemaker is being inserted, the atrial pacing wire will be placed in the right atrial appendage (8). If the pacemaker is being inserted by the patient's bedside without the aid of fluoroscopy, a pulmonary artery balloon flotation catheter can be used to float the pacing wires into position. These catheters have two pacing ports, so they can be used for dual-chamber pacing (8).

Once the pacing wire(s) are in position, they are attached to the external pacemaker and the stimulation threshold is measured. To do this, set the pacing rate at 5–10 beats per minute faster than the patient's rate, and set the milliamperage at 5 mA and turn the milliamperage down in 1-mA increments until the pacing fails. This is the pacing/stimulation threshold (6). Generally, the lower the pacing threshold, the better the contact between the electrode and the endocardium (13). Acceptable stimulation thresholds are below 1 volt, although higher levels may be acceptable if the patient is elderly, has had an inferior infarct or if several sites have been tried, all with relatively high thresholds (9). The stability of the pacing wire is then checked by pacing, at an output of twice the stimulation

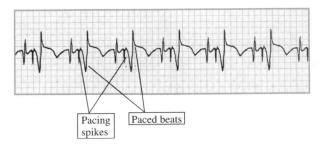

Pacing spikes   Paced beats

Figure 10.1. ECG of paced beats.

threshold, during deep breathing. If capture is lost during this manoeuvre, then a more stable position will be found (9).

Finally, the pacing wire will be sutured firmly to the skin. A loop will be formed on the chest wall to minimise the chance of accidentally dislodging the lead (9). A self-adhesive, semi-permeable, transparent dressing should be applied over the sheath entry site. The nurse should record the time and date and whenever the dressing has been changed (8).

After placement of the temporary pacemaker is completed, a chest x-ray should be taken to locate the placement of the lead, and to exclude a pneumothorax when the internal jugular or subclavian vein is used for access (1).

A 12-lead electrocardiogram (ECG) of the paced complexes should always be examined to ensure correlation with presumed position of the catheter. Instead of a P wave, a narrow, bright, vertical line, referred to as a pacing spike, should be seen on the ECG (see Figure 10.1). There should be no equivalent of P–R gap on the ECG, as the pacing wire is in direct contact with the myocardial tissue. Pacing from the typical right ventricular apical position should produce a large, wide left-bundle branch block pattern and should have a consistent shape (4). Pacing from the left ventricle (via a septal defect, for example), in the cardiac veins or in the pericardial space will yield a different QRS morphology (1).

A LOOK AT A PULSE GENERATOR

The pulse generator of a temporary pacemaker is a device that sits outside the body. It contains several controls that regulate the current output, heart rate and sensitivity, and the mode of pacing. If a temporary dual chamber pacemaker is being used, it will have separate terminals for the atrial and ventricular inputs. The wires should be labelled appropriately, indicating whether they are pacing the atrium or the ventricle. Care should be taken not to interchange these leads when attaching them to the pulse generator (8). Figure 10.2 is an illustration of a single-chamber temporary pulse generator, with brief descriptions of its various parts.

Depending on the manufacturer, temporary pacemakers may look different, but there are three control buttons whose setting should be checked at least daily: rate, stimulation threshold and sensitivity threshold.

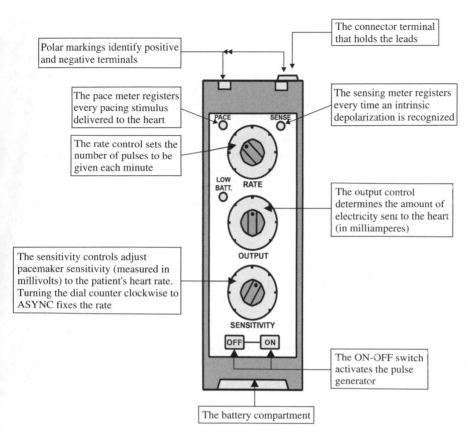

Figure 10.2. A temporary pacemaker.

Rate

The rate control regulates how many impulses are generated in 1 minute and is measured in pulses per minute (ppm). The rate is usually set between 60 and 80 ppm. The pacemaker fires if the patient's heart rate falls below the preset rate. The rate may be higher if the patient has a tachyarrhythmia and is being treated with overdrive pacing (3).

Stimulation threshold

The stimulation threshold is the least amount of electrical energy required for the cardiac muscle to depolarise/contract consistently (3). This is sometimes referred to as the pacing threshold (8). For temporary pacemakers, this energy is measured in milliamperes (mA) (8). If the electrode is positioned adequately, the stimulation threshold should be less than 1.5 mA. However, the stimulation threshold can increase or decrease within hours of placing the electrode (13). Factors that affect stimulation threshold include hypoxia, electrolyte imbalance (e.g. hypokalaemia), antidysrhythmic drugs, catecholamines, digoxin toxicity and corticosteroids (8).

Therefore, the stimulation threshold should be checked at least twice a day or per shift, depending on hospital protocol, as a sudden increase in the stimulation threshold usually indicates that the electrodes need to be repositioned (8; 9). The steps for checking the stimulation threshold are as follows:

1. Give a brief explanation to the patient.
2. Ensure that the patient is in a paced rhythm. This may mean temporarily increasing the pacing rate to override the patient's intrinsic rhythm for the procedure (14).
3. Whilst observing the cardiac monitor, gradually reduce the energy output of the pulse generator, until a pacing spike appears but is not followed by an appropriate wave form (8).
4. This is referred to as loss of capture (14).
5. Gradually turn up the output until a QRS complex follows each pacing spike. The amount of current used when 1:1 capture first occurs is the stimulation threshold (14). The mA threshold, then, is the number on which the dial is set at that time.
6. Once the threshold has been ascertained, the output voltage should be set at three times the threshold to ensure a margin of safety. For example, if the consistent capture is regained at 2 mA, the output should be set for 6 mA (9).
7. If the rate has been temporarily increased for testing purposes, decrease it to the ordered rate.
8. Document mA of the stimulation threshold and the final mA setting used (8).

Sensitivity threshold

Pacemakers can work in two modes. The first mode is asynchronous, also known as a fixed-rate pacemaker, which will pace the heart at a set rhythm, no matter what the heart's own rhythm might be (3). This mode is rarely used, as sometimes it can result in a life-threatening arrhythmia, such as ventricular fibrillation, if the patient's own intrinsic rhythm resumes (4).

The second mode is synchronous, or a demand pacemaker, which senses the heart's own intrinsic rhythm and paces only when the heart cannot generate an electrical impulse faster than the lowest rate set on the pacemaker. This mode allows the heart rhythm to resume naturally as it recovers its conduction potential (4).

The sensitivity threshold is the smallest amount of electrical activity generated by the heart that the pacemaker will sense and then inhibit its own impulse generation (8). The heart's own electrical impulses are measured in millivolts (8). When a synchronous pacemaker senses a preset level of millivolts, it will inhibit the next pacing stimulus and reset the pacing interval (14). The higher the number of millivolts that the pacemaker is set to, the larger the heart's own intrinsic heart beat must be to generate enough millivolts for the pacemaker to sense them. When the pacemaker's sensitivity needs to be increased to enable the pacemaker to 'see' smaller signals from the heart, the sensitivity setting has to be decreased (14).

If the sensitivity setting is too high on the pacemaker, undersensing occurs. However, when the pacemaker is set to the most sensitive setting, the pacemaker could sense extraneous signals, such as T wave or signals from the other chambers in the heart, and oversensing occurs (8).

The sensitivity threshold of a pacemaker can only be ascertained if the patient has a stable underlying rhythm. If the patient is completely pacemaker-dependent or has a very slow underlying rate, do not perform a sensitivity threshold test (14). The procedure for performing a sensitivity threshold test is as follows:

1. Give a brief explanation to the patient.
2. Verify that the patient has intrinsic rhythm. This may require decreasing the pacing rate temporarily to assess the underlying rhythm (14).
3. Slowly reduce the pacemaker's sensitivity by increasing the number on the sensitivity control (14).
4. Observe the sense indicator light and the cardiac monitor:
   (a) The sensing indicator light should flash with each sensed P wave for atrial pacing, or QRS for ventricular pacing (14).
   (b) Pacing will remain inhibited and there are no pacing spikes seen on the monitor as long as sensing continues (14).
5. Note when the sense indicator fails to flash with each P wave or QRS and when pacing spikes begin to appear in competition with the intrinsic rhythm. This is the sensitivity threshold (14).
6. Set the sensitivity setting at half the identified threshold to ensure an adequate safety margin. For example, if the sensitivity threshold is 5 mV, set the sensitivity setting at 2.5 mV (14).
7. Return the pacing rate setting back to the ordered rate.
8. Document the sensitivity threshold and final setting (8).

WHAT TO OBSERVE FOR WHEN A PATIENT HAS A TEMPORARY PACEMAKER IN SITU

Following a temporary pacemaker insertion, a nurse should be vigilant in observing for potential complications and malfunction of a temporary pacemaker. Although temporary transvenous pacing is an invasive but relatively simple procedure, complications are common because it is often carried out by inexperienced, unsupervised operators (2). Complications encountered include the following.

Pneumothorax

After any subclavian venous puncture, a chest x-ray should be requested to check for a pneumothorax. In patients with severe respiratory disease, in whom a pneumothorax might provoke respiratory failure, alternative pacing routes should be considered (7).

Subclavian artery puncture

Even in the most experienced hands, it is possible to puncture the subclavian artery rather than the subclavian vein. If arterial puncture should occur, serious consequences are rare. The exception, however, is in thrombolysed patients, in whom severe bleeding may result. Unfortunately, the position of the subclavian artery makes it difficult to apply pressure; therefore, bleeding may be difficult to control. For this reason, where possible, the subclavian vein should be avoided when temporary pacing becomes necessary following thrombolysis in acute myocardial infarction. Venous access for pacing can also be achieved by the antecubital veins, the femoral vein or the jugular vein (7).

Lead perforation

Occasionally, the electrode tip may perforate the thin right ventricular myocardium (2). This may occur acutely during lead positioning or due to gradual erosion over a number of days. It causes a rise in the threshold and may result in loss of pacing. The threshold should be checked every day in a patient with a temporary wire to detect any change in the threshold which might indicate perforation (7). If the pacing lead perforates the septum and enters the left ventricle, the ECG may show a right bundle branch pattern rather than the usual left bundle branch pattern (14). When perforation occurs, it may result in failure to pace, diaphragmatic stimulation, pericardial friction rub and pericardial pain and may, occasionally, cause cardiac tamponade (2).

Hiccups/muscle twitching

If the patient hiccups in synchrony with their pacing spike, this can indicate that they are pacing their phrenic nerve as a result of an excessively high output setting (13). Other causes include perforation of the cardiac wall and pacing wire dislodgement (3), and a crack in the pacing wire can cause pacing of the pectoral muscles (11).

Exit block

Sometimes, pacing failure occurs without electrode tip displacement or another cause. In these cases, failure is attributed to 'exit block', which is caused by excessive tissue reaction at the junction between the electrode tip and the endocardium (2). Therefore, the pacing threshold should be checked at least daily and the voltage increased if necessary (11).

Infection

The patient's temperature should be checked at least four times a day, as pyrexia indicates that they have developed an infection. Blood cultures should be taken and the patient started on intravenous antibiotics. The temporary pacemaker should be removed. If the patient still requires temporary pacing, another pacing wire should be inserted via another route prior to its removal (11).

TROUBLESHOOTING MALFUNCTIONS OF TEMPORARY PACEMAKERS

In addition to these potential complications to the patient, problems with the pulse generator itself, the leads and the connections should be observed for. Temporary pacemaker malfunctions in a pacemaker-dependent patient can lead to a medical emergency because without an effective underlying rhythm, the patient may be asystolic or severely symptomatic because of a slow, ineffective heart rate (14). Drug therapy (atropine), cardiac pulmonary resuscitation and transcutaneous pacing may be required until the cause of the problem is found and corrected (8).

Some of the more common problems encountered with temporary pacemakers include the following.

Failure to discharge

When the pacemaker fires, it appears as a tall, narrow wave on the ECG, referred to as a 'pacing spike' (Figure 10.1). Failure to discharge results in absence of the pacing spike and unexplained loss of pacing. The cause of this failure may be with the pulse generator itself – either the processor or battery failure (8). The batteries should be changed first and if that does not work, the pulse generator should be replaced (8).

A lead/electrode fracture will not have a pacing spike on the ECG, so should be considered if the above measures do not resolve the problem (2). This may result from kinking of the wire. A complete fracture may be detected by chest x-ray, and the lead will have to be replaced (11).

Failure to capture

Failure to capture is indicated on an ECG by a pacing spike without the appropriate atrial or ventricular response, namely a pacing spike not followed by an appropriate waveform (3). Causes include a low output setting, depletion of the battery, an electrolyte imbalance or an increase in pacing threshold from medication or metabolic changes, acidosis, fibrosis around the tip of the wire, a broken or cracked lead wire, an incorrect lead position or perforation of the lead through the myocardium (3; 8).

As all temporary pacemaker malfunctions should be checked in a systematic manner, the following steps should be followed:

1. Increase pulse generator output (in milliamperes) to the highest setting, asynchronous mode.
2. Check all connections.
3. Replace pulse generator or battery; be prepared for transcutaneous pacing backup during the change.
4. Inform the medical staff (8).

Undersensing

Failure of the pacemaker to sense intrinsic beats is known as undersensing (8). It can be identified on the ECG by pacing spikes appearing where they should not. Although they can appear in any part of the cardiac cycle, pacing spikes are especially dangerous if they fall on the T wave, as they can cause ventricular tachycardia or fibrillation (8).

The most likely cause of sensing failure in the temporary pacemaker is lead displacement. However, pulse generator failure, lead insulation defect or lead wire fracture may also cause undersensing (3).

To correct undersensing problems in the temporary pacemaker:

1. First, ascertain that the lead is properly connected to the temporary pacemaker.
2. If all the connections are in place, increase the sensitivity of the pacemaker by turning the dial to a lower millivolt value.
3. If problems persist, inform medical staff, as the leads may need to be repositioned (8).
4. Turning the patient on their left side sometimes temporarily works when the pacing wire loses contact with the ventricle (14).

Oversensing

Oversensing means that the pacemaker is so sensitive that it inappropriately senses internal or external signals as QRS complexes and inhibits its output (14). This means that the pacemaker will not pace when the patient actually needs it, so becomes symptomatic (3). Internal sources that cause oversensing include tall T or P waves being mistaken for QRS complexes (8). External sources can be electromagnetic or radio-frequency signals from electronic equipment near the pacemaker, such as an electrical razor or toothbrush. Oversensing is usually due to the sensitivity being set too high (14). However, electrode displacement or impending lead fracture may cause oversensing. A partially fractured lead often allows signals to saturate the pulse generator, causing oversensing and inhibiting the pacing output in demand mode (8).

To correct the oversensing problem in a temporary pacemaker:

1. First, turn the sensitivity control down.
2. Check all the connections.
3. Change the battery or pulse generator.
4. Remove items from the room that might cause electromagnetic interference.
5. If the bed is electronic, check that it is grounded.
6. Unplug each piece of equipment, and then see whether the interference has stopped.
7. If the pacemaker still fires on the *T* wave, turn off the pacemaker (with the permission of the doctor). Ensure that atropine and transcutaneous pacing are easily available in case the patient's heart rate drops (3).

WHAT TO DO WHEN THE TEMPORARY PACEMAKER MALFUNCTIONS

Potential problem	Nursing/medical action
The pacemaker setting has been altered by the patient or somebody else	1. Return the pacemaker setting to the correct position 2. Ensure that the protective plastic shield is covering the pacemaker dials Remind the patient that only staff members should adjust the dials on the pacemaker unit (3)
Output setting is too low	Increase the milliamperes setting slowly according to your unit's policy (3)
Broken connection	Check all the connections (8)
Battery is low	Change the battery (3)
Pulse generator is not working properly	Change the pulse generator (3)
Changes in metabolism/medications may increase the stimulation threshold	1. Increase the milliamperes until capture is maintained (8) 2. Check the urea and electrolytes and correct the metabolic imbalance (8) 3. Review patient medication (3)
Lead dislodgement/pacing wire is not in contact with the myocardium	1. Obtain a chest x-ray to confirm 2. This can sometimes be temporarily corrected by repositioning the patient on their left side (8; 14)

Potential problem	Nursing/medical action
	3. The lead will have to be repositioned by medical staff (8)
Lead fracture	1. Obtain a chest x-ray to confirm 2. The lead will have to be replaced by medical staff (8)
The pulse generator is oversensing	1. Reduce the sensitivity setting on the control by increasing the millivolts 2. If the patient is pacer-dependent (no intrinsic R wave), change the program to asynchronous mode until the problem has been identified 3. Identify the cause of the oversensing (8)
The oversensing is caused by cross-talk in a dual chamber pacemaker The pulse generator detects signals for the other chamber and inhibits its output	1. If the atrial channel misinterprets the R wave as a P wave, the sensitivity of the atrial channel should be reduced (8) 2. If the ventricular channel misinterprets the atrial pacing spike as an R wave, it will inappropriately inhibit its impulse. The output (mA) from the atrial channel should be reduced and the ventricular channel sensitivity should be decreased by increasing the mV setting
A crack in the insulation around the wire may result in current leakage to the pectoral muscle touching the pacing wire	Signs include intermittent pacing and a reduced amplitude due to the loss of current to the myocardium (11) 1. Increase the milliamperes until capture is maintained 2. The lead will have to be replaced by medical staff (8)
Perforation of the lead wire through the myocardium	Signs include a decrease in blood pressure and an increase in sinus rate (8) 1. Obtain an echocardiogram to confirm (8) 2. The lead will have to be replaced by medical staff (8)

Potential problem	Nursing/medical action
Delivery of a pacing during the ventricles' refractory period when the heart is physiologically unable to respond to the stimulus	This problem occurs with loss of sensing (undersensing) and can be prevented by correcting the sensing problem (14)

CARE PLANS

PROBLEM/NEED

Patient requires a temporary pacing wire

PRE-IMPLANT ACTION

Goal/aim of care

The nursing care is directed towards preparing the patient for temporary pacemaker insertion, ensuring pre, peri and post-procedure safety.

Action	Rationale
If time permits, provide appropriate explanations and information to both the patient and family members	Being informed about a procedure reduces anxiety levels in patients and their families (5)
Ensure that a working temporary pulse generator is available	The pacemaker box should be checked prior to use to ensure that it is working correctly (9)
Insert a new battery in the pulse generator (date of battery change should be noted on the pacemaker box)	To ensure that the pulse generator is working correctly (9)
Ensure that the patient has a patent peripheral intravenous cannula	Venous access is important to administer emergency drugs during the procedure, if required (4; 9)
Shave the skin in the area that the doctor intends to insert the pacing wire	Body hair is removed in order to reduce infection risk during the procedure (14)
Ensure that identification and allergy bands are correct, legible and secure	To ensure correct identification and prevent possible problems (14)

Action	Rationale
Obtain baseline blood pressure, pulse, temperature, respiration rate and blood glucose	In order to provide a baseline, for comparison after the pacemaker has been inserted (4)
If the patient's clinical condition permits, record a 12-lead ECG	In order to provide a baseline, for comparison after the pacemaker has been inserted (4)

NURSING ACTION IF ASSISTING AT THE BEDSIDE OR IN THE FLUOROSCOPY SUITE

Action	Rationale
Collect equipment: a. Skin preparation solutions, such as those with an iodine base b. Local anaesthetic (lidocaine, 1 or 2%) c. Pacer catheter that has been selected by the physician d. Alligator clamps e. Bridging cable f. Percutaneous introducer or 14-gauge needle g. Sterile dressings (either gauze or transparent) and tape h. Sterile towels i. Masks and sterile gowns and gloves j. Cut-down tray, if needed k. Suture with needle (silk generally used)	To ensure that what is required during the procedure is available (13)
Ensure that resuscitation equipment is easily accessible	Resuscitation equipment should be accessible because when the pacing wire passes through the tricuspid valve, ventricular arrhythmias may be induced (4; 9)
Ensure that a transcutaneous pacemaker is easily accessible	In case the patient requires temporary short-term pacing support until the transvenous pacemaker is in place (9)

Action	Rationale
Have emergency drugs ready for use: lidocaine, atropine and isoproterenol	Brady or tachyarrhythmias are often induced during the procedure (9)
Sedate the patient, if necessary	To reduce anxiety and make them more comfortable (13)
Attach the ECG machine to the patient	In order to monitor the cardiac rhythm closely throughout the procedure; inform the physician of any arrhythmias or ventricular irritability (13)
Attach the blood pressure cuff and oxygen saturation monitor to the patient	Blood pressure should be observed every 10–15 minutes or more frequently if the patient is symptomatic (13). A decrease in oxygen saturations may indicate a pneumothorax
The area selected for insertion of the pacing wire should be cleaned using a skin preparation solution such as alcoholic providone 10% which is allowed to dry. Then, the surgical drapes are applied around the area	In order to maintain asepsis (12)
Check the level of local anaesthesia with the patient. Is the patient feeling any pain?	To ensure that the patient is anaesthetised properly prior to inserting the percutaneous sheath (13)
Provide reassurance throughout the procedure	If the patient is experiencing a symptomatic bradycardia and feeling extremely unwell, they will appreciate some friendly reassurance (4)

NURSING CARE POST TEMPORARY PACEMAKER INSERTION

Action	Rationale
Attach the patient to a cardiac monitor	There should be continuous monitoring for at least the first 24 hours to ensure that the temporary pacemaker is working normally (4)

Action	Rationale
Obtain an ECG	For baseline determination of lead position (1)
Check the stimulation threshold	The stimulation threshold is the current necessary to consistently induce the ventricles to contract. On warding, this should be recorded to obtain a baseline. Then it should be checked twice daily (4)
Check the sensitivity	The sensitivity threshold senses the patient's intrinsic heart beat. This should be checked and recorded initially and if the patient is not completely pacemaker-dependent, at least once every 24 hours (13)
Check the rate	The rate regulates how many impulses are generated in 1 minute. This should be checked and recorded (3)
Check the mode of the pacemaker	Record whether it is an asynchronous (fixed) or synchronous (demand) pacemaker (13)
Obtain a chest x-ray, which should be checked by medical staff	1. To ensure the pacing wire's position and 2. To check for pneumothorax if the internal jugular or subclavian vein puncture was used (1)
Electively restrict the patient's motion to prevent pacer wire dislodgment	a. Antecubital approach: an arm board should be used to immobilise the arm. The pulse generator is secured on the arm with either gauze, an elastic bandage or specially made Velcro straps for this purpose. Padding around the elbow as well as underneath the pacemaker box usually prevents pressure sores from developing. Abduction of the patient's arm is prevented by positioning the patient with pillows in bed or securing the arm to the body with an elastic wrap or gauze bandage if the patient is sitting up or

Action	Rationale
	ambulating. If the patient is oriented and cooperative, these last measures may not be necessary. If the pacemaker is one of the older models, the area of connection between the terminal pacer wires and the pacemaker box should be covered with a nonconductive material, such as a rubber glove, for added precaution. The extremities should be elevated slightly with a pillow to facilitate venous return, and pulses should be checked distally to determine adequacy of circulation (13)
	b. Femoral approach: usually, a bridging cable (extension) is used between the terminal ends of the catheter and the pulse generator. The pulse generator is fastened to the thigh area, but, for the patient's comfort (because of its weight), it may be better carried around the waist by using an elastic bandage, gauze or specially designed Velcro belt. If wearing the pulse generator around the waist is not satisfactory for the patient, the pacer box is placed in a cloth bag and suspended on an IV pole on or adjacent to the bed (13)
	c. Jugular or subclavian approach: an extension cable is used, and the pulse generator is attached at the patient's waist or on an IV pole adjacent to or on the bed (13)
Enforce bed rest initially as per the doctor's advice	Physician's advice varies in opinion regarding increased activity (13)
Administer an analgesic, as needed, for comfort	The patient may experience some local discomfort, particularly if a cut-down was necessary (13)

Action	Rationale
Document the following: a. Date and time of insertion b. Type of wire inserted and location of insertion c. Mode of action (i.e. demand or fixed-rate) d. Whether the pacer is on or off e. Rate setting of pacer (pulses per minute) f. Threshold level and mA setting (for AV sequential pacing, both atrial and ventricular milliamperes need to be recorded) g. Millivolts on sensitivity dial h. AV interval (in milliseconds) if AV sequential mode is used	This is good clinical practice and enables nursing/medical staff on different shifts to: 1. check the thresholds, because if these change, it can indicate a problem with the pacemaker or leads 2. check that people are not interfering with the pulse generator (13)
Check and document stimulation threshold twice a day	A sudden increase in the stimulation threshold can indicate: 1. that the electrodes need to be repositioned (8) 2. cardiac perforation (7)
Attach a monitor rhythm strip to the chart at least every 4 hours	In order to measure the rate and automatic interval to confirm that the pacemaker is functioning properly (13)
Observe for signs of haematoma	If the patient has undergone thrombolysis for an acute myocardial infarction, this increases the risk of bleeding at the puncture site. Therefore, frequent checks for haematoma should be made (4)
Check body temperature every 4 hours	To assess for signs of infection (4)
During dressing change, watch for any signs of infection or cellulitis	People with a temporary pacemaker are at increased risk of infection; therefore, the insertion site should be checked for any redness, swelling, drainage, unusual tenderness, warmth and pain. Document your observations (13)

Action	Rationale
Be aware of the patient's electrolyte status, especially the serum potassium level, throughout the pacing period	The pacemaker threshold is lower in the presence of electrolyte imbalance (e.g. hypokalaemia) (3; 13)
Be aware of safety precautions	a. Anyone handling exposed lead wires should wear rubber gloves b. The junction between the temporary lead and the pulse generator should be protected, and uninsulated portions of the pacing lead should be covered c. Check all connections (wire to bridging cable, cable to pulse generator) daily d. Keep dressing over the pacing wire insertion sites dry, as wet dressings conduct electricity (8; 14)
Be careful when repositioning patients with temporary pacemakers	Turning may dislodge the pacing lead (3)

REFERENCES

1. Baim, D. S. and Grossman, W. (2000) *Grossman's Cardiac Catheterization: Angiography, and Intervention*, 6th edn, London, Lippincott Williams & Wilkins.
2. Bennett, D. H. (2002) *Cardiac Arrhythmias: Practical Notes on Interpretation and Treatment*, London, Arnold.
3. Beverage, D., Haworth, K., Labus, D., Mayer, B. and Munson, S. (2005) *ECG Interpretation Made Incredibly Easy*, London, Lippincott Williams & Wilkins.
4. Hubbard, J. (2003) 'An overview of permanent and temporary cardiac pacemakers', *Nursing Times*, **99**(36): 26–7.
5. Hughes, S. (2002) 'The effects of pre-operative information', *Nursing Standard*, **16**: 28, 33–7.
6. Kern, M. (2003) *The Cardiac Catheterisation Handbook*, 4th edn, London, Mosby.
7. Julian, D. G., Cowan, J. C. and McLenachan, J. M. (2005) *Cardiology*, 8th edn, Edinburgh, Elsevier Saunders Co. Ltd.
8. Morton, P., Fontaine, D., Hudak, C. and Gallo, B. (2005) *Critical Care Nursing: A Holistic Approach*, 8th edn, Philadelphia, PA, Lippincott Williams & Wilkins.
9. Nolan, J., Greenwood, J. and Mackintosh, A. (1998) *Cardiac Emergencies: A Pocket Guide*, Oxford, Butterworth Heinemann.
10. Rosendorff, C. (2005) *Essential Cardiology: Principles and Practice*, 2nd edn, Totowa, NJ, Humana Press.

11. Swanton, R. (2003) *Cardiology*, 5th edn, Oxford, Blackwell Science.
12. Thompson, P. L. (1997) *Coronary Care Manual*, London, Churchill Livingstone.
13. Woods, S., Froelicher, E. and Motzer, S. (1997) *Cardiac Nursing*, 3rd edn, Philadelphia, PA, Lippincott Williams & Wilkins.
14. Woods, S., Froelicher, E. and Motzer, S. (2000) *Cardiac Nursing*, 4th edn, Philadelphia, PA, Lippincott Williams & Wilkins.

11   Permanent Pacemakers

CONDUCTION IN THE HEART

The heart is a muscular pump, composed of four chambers that work in conjunction with each other. The top two chambers, called the right and left atria, serve as volume reservoirs for blood being sent to the bottom two chambers, called the right and left ventricles. When the atria contract, they force blood into the relaxed ventricles. The ventricles serve as the pumping chambers of the heart and when the two ventricles contract, they force the blood to the lungs and the body, while the relaxed atria fill up with blood, and the cycle begins again (3; 22).

The heart cannot pump unless an electrical stimulus occurs first. The sinoatrial node (SA node) is the heart's main pacemaker, and automatically generates electrical impulses 60–100 times per minute. When initiated, the impulse follows a specific path through the heart, called the conduction system. Impulses that form in the SA node travel through the Bachmann's bundle, which are tracts of tissue extending from the sinus node to the left atrium. Impulses are thought to be transmitted through the right atrium via intra-nodal tracts. Impulse transmission through the right and left atria occurs so rapidly that the atria contract almost simultaneously (3; 22) (see Figure 11.1).

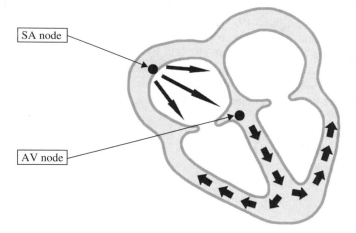

Figure 11.1. Picture of heart showing normal conduction.

The band of tissue that separates the atria from the ventricles is non-conductable and the impulse is transmitted to the ventricles via the atrioventricular node (AV node). The AV node's main function is to delay the impulses by 0.04 seconds to keep the ventricles from contracting too quickly. This delay allows the ventricles to complete their filling phase as the atria contract (3; 22).

The impulse is transmitted next to the bundle of His, which is a tract of tissue that extends into the ventricles next to the interventricular septum. The bundle eventually splits into right and left bundle branches which transmit the impulse to the right and left ventricles, initiating them to contract simultaneously. To assist the conduction across the ventricles, fibres known as Purkinje fibres extend from the bundle branches into the endocardium, deep into the myocardial tissue. The entire network of specialised nervous tissue that extends through the ventricles is known as the His–Purkinje system (3; 22).

An interruption in the conduction system may impede the heart's ability to pump efficiently and may be life-threatening. In order to restore conduction, a pacemaker may be required.

WHAT IS A PACEMAKER?

A pacemaker is defined as a battery-operated generator that initiates and controls the electrical stimulation of the heart via one or more electrodes that are in direct contact with the myocardium (10). If the heart beats too slowly, too quickly or irregularly, a patient may become symptomatic and thus require a pacemaker (23).

The pacemaker system consists of the pacemaker itself (also referred to as a pulse generator) and wires (also referred to as leads/electrodes) that connect the pacemaker to the heart (9). The pacemaker is composed of a lithium iodide battery source and micro-computer circuits enclosed in a hermetically sealed metal container. The generator weighs 20–30 grams and is 5–7 mm thick (15). The pulse generator is typically described as being slightly larger than a man's wristwatch. Usually, only a small bump in the skin is seen over the place where the pacemaker has been implanted. The computer circuits perform the functions of monitoring the patient's underlying heart rhythm and delivering an electrical impulse which causes the heart to beat at the desired rate. Many pacemakers implanted today also may have rate-responsiveness features that allow pacing of the heart at faster rates during periods of exercise (24).

Pacemakers fall into two categories – synchronous and asynchronous – based on how they stimulate the heart:

> A *synchronous* or '*on-demand*' pacemaker continuously monitors the patient's intrinsic heart rhythm and paces when the heart cannot generate an electrical impulse faster than the slowest rate set on the pacemaker. This method allows the heart to take over when normal conduction is restored (10).

An *asynchronous* or *'fixed rate'* pacemaker fires at a fixed heart rate and does not monitor the heart's intrinsic heart rhythm. The disadvantage of this method is that competition between the paced beat and the patient's intrinsic rhythm may occur when normal conduction is re-established, sometimes resulting in life-threatening arrhythmias such as ventricular fibrillation (10).

The pacing leads are flexible, insulated wires with one or two electrodes at each tip (9). The electrodes not only deliver the electrical stimuli to the myocardium, but they are also able to sense spontaneous electrical activity from the heart (1). The pacing leads can be affixed to the myocardium with a lead-fixation device, called active fixation. These devices include screws or coils. Another alternative is to use passives (tines) and steroid-eluting electrodes (tips designed to reduce cardiac inflammation). Over time, fibrous tissue forms around the tip of the lead to secure its placement and ensure proper function of the electrode (15).

WHO NEEDS A PERMANENT PACEMAKER?

Although the majority of pacemakers are inserted when the heart beats too slowly (bradycardia), they are also inserted for some conditions in which the heart beats too quickly (tachycardia) or irregularly (23). In addition to this, with advances in pacemaker technology, they are now being used to treat patients with class III and IV heart failure. For these patients, both ventricles are paced, so it is known as biventricular pacing or cardiac resynchronisation therapy (3).

The following is a list of specific indications for insertion of a permanent pacemaker, which will be discussed in more detail.

Indications for permanent pacing:

- brady-arrhythmias;
- sick sinus syndrome;
- following anterior myocardial infarction (MI) and necrosis of the conduction system;
- atrial fibrillation (AF) with a slow ventricular response;
- atrioventricular (AV) heart block;
- congenital heart block;
- tachyarrhythmias when drug therapy is ineffective may be combined with an automatic implantable cardioverter defibrillator;
- management of chronic heart failure (10).

BRADYCARDIA

The most common reason for pacemaker implantation is because the sinus node function becomes too slow from age, heart disease or medications (24). At rest, the heart usually beats about 50–70 beats per minute, and the heart rate may

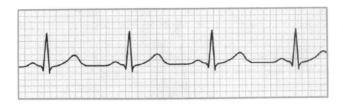

Figure 11.2. ECG strip of sinus bradycardia.

increase two to threefold during exercise or stress (24). Sinus bradycardia is characterised by a sinus rate below 60 beats per minute and is regular (see Figure 11.2). Sinus bradycardia itself is rarely an indication for pacing in the absence of symptoms. Highly trained athletes often have baseline heart rates in the 40s or even in the 30s (2), and sinus bradycardia can also occur normally during sleep due to decreased metabolic demands (3).

However, when sinus bradycardia produces symptoms, prompt attention is critical, as the patient might not be able to compensate for a drop in heart rate by increasing their stroke volume. As a result, the brain and body do not get enough blood flow and a variety of symptoms may result, such as fainting (syncope), near fainting, dizziness, lack of energy, shortness of breath and exercise intolerance (24). In addition, bradycardia also disposes some patients to more serious arrhythmias, such as ventricular tachycardia (VT) and ventricular fibrillation (3).

SICK SINUS SYNDROME

Sick sinus syndrome is also called sinus nodal dysfunction and sinoatrial disease, and refers to a wide spectrum of sinus-node abnormalities. The syndrome is caused by a disturbance in the way in which impulses are generated or the inability to conduct impulses in the atrium (3). It is one of the most common causes of profound symptomatic bradycardia; a good example is when the sinus node fails to generate an adequate heart rate (2).

Patients with sick sinus syndrome are prone to attacks of atrial tachyarrhythmias, such as AF, atrial flutter or ectopic atrial tachycardia – a condition sometimes referred to as bradycardia–tachycardia (or brady–tachy) syndrome (3). It is believed that the long pauses which result in profound bradycardia, which usually occur after the termination of an attack of a tachyarrhythmia, are due to a prolonged recovery time of the sinus-node function. This may result in severe light-headedness or syncope at the time of conversion from the rapid rhythm (2). In addition to this, the prolonged periods of sinus arrest, in which the atria are not moving, increase the patient's risk of developing systemic emboli, resulting in stroke, pulmonary or peripheral embolisation (20).

MYOCARDIAL INFARCTION

The need for permanent pacing after acute MI is related to the site of the MI, its extent and the type of block that it may cause. The need for temporary pacing during the acute phase of an MI is not in itself an indication for permanent pacing (2).

Following an inferior MI, second to third-degree AV block is normally transient, and permanent pacing does not need to be considered for 2–3 weeks post infarct. Following an anterior MI, complete AV block usually represents massive septal necrosis, and mortality from left-ventricle failure is high. Persistent complete AV block is permanently paced. It is more difficult to decide whether an AV block that regresses during hospital stay needs a permanent pacemaker. This is still a subject for debate, but 24-hour Holter monitoring may help to identify subjects at risk who need permanent pacing. The ventricular myocardium is often very irritable in the post-infarct period and, if possible, permanent pacing should be avoided in the first 3–4 weeks (20).

ATRIAL FIBRILLATION WITH SLOW VENTRICULAR RESPONSE

Atrial fibrillation is defined as chaotic, asynchronous, electrical activity in atrial tissue (see Figure 11.3). It stems from the firing of a number of impulses in circus re-entry pathways; the ectopic impulses may fire at a rate of 400–600 times per minute, causing the atria to quiver rather than contract, resulting in the loss of atrial kick. The ventricles respond only to those impulses that make it through the AV node (3). If the resulting ventricular response is too slow, there will be a drop in cardiac output, producing symptoms such as dizziness, shortness of breath and poor exertional tolerance, so a pacemaker is indicated (10).

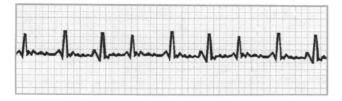

Figure 11.3. ECG strip of atrial fibrillation.

ATRIO-VENTRICULAR BLOCK

The other leading cause for pacemaker implantation is failure of the normal electrical signal to reach the main pumping chambers, causing a slow heart rate known as heart block (24). Atrioventricular heart block results from an interruption in the conduction of impulses between the atria and the ventricles. Atrioventricular block can be total or partial, or it may delay conduction. The block can occur at the AV node, the bundle of His or the bundle branches (3). The clinical effect of the block depends on how the impulses are blocked, how slow the ventricular rate is as a result and how the block ultimately affects the heart. A slow ventricular rate can decrease cardiac output, possibly causing light-headedness, hypotension and confusion (3).

Atrioventricular blocks are classified according to their severity, not their location. That severity is measured according to how well the node conducts impulses and the blocks are called first, second and third-degree blocks (3).

First-degree AV block occurs when the impulses from the atria are consistently delayed during conduction through the AV node (see Figure 11.4). Conduction eventually occurs; it just takes longer than normal. The presence of first-degree block is the least dangerous type of AV block, and indicates some kind of problem in the conduction system, so should be monitored to ensure that it has not developed into a more severe block. As most patients with first-degree block show no symptoms because cardiac output is not significantly affected, any underlying causes are treated, but a pacemaker is not required (3).

Second-degree AV block is also known as Mobitz block, and falls into two categories. Type I second-degree AV block, also known as Wenckebach block, occurs when each successive impulse from the SA node is delayed slightly longer than the previous impulse. The pattern continues until an impulse fails to be conducted to the ventricles, and the cycle then repeats. Type I second-degree block may occur normally in an otherwise healthy person. It is almost always temporary, and usually resolves when the underlying condition is corrected, so does not need a pacemaker (3).

Type II second-degree AV block is less common than type I, but is more serious. It occurs when occasional impulses from the SA node fail to conduct to the ventricles (see Figure 11.5). This block is more serious than type I, as the ventricular rate tends to be slower and the cardiac output diminished, and it is therefore more likely to cause symptoms. Usually, chronic type II AV block may progress to complete heart block, so requires a pacemaker (3).

Third-degree heart block, also known as complete heart block, occurs when impulses from the atria are completely blocked at the AV node and cannot be

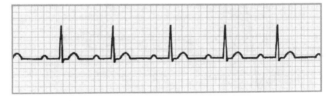

Figure 11.4. ECG strip showing first-degree block.

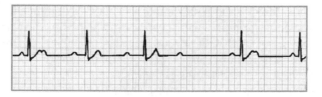

Figure 11.5. ECG strip showing second-degree block.

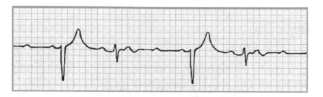

Figure 11.6. ECG strip showing complete heart block.

conducted to the ventricles (see Figure 11.6). Acting independently, the atria are generally under the control of the SA node, and tend to maintain a regular rate of 60–100 beats per minute. The ventricular rhythm can originate from the AV node itself and maintain a rate of 40–60 beats per minute. Most typically, it originates from the Purkinje system in the ventricle and maintains a rate of 20–40 beats per minute (3).

Because the ventricular rate is so slow, third-degree AV block presents a potentially life-threatening situation because cardiac output can drop dramatically. Most patients with third-degree AV block experience significant symptoms, including severe fatigue, dyspnoea, chest pain, light-headedness, changes in mental status and loss of consciousness. Signs include hypotension, pallor, diaphoresis, bradycardia and a variation in the intensity of the pulse. A permanent block requires a permanent pacemaker (3).

Without pacing, the prognosis in patients with complete heart block is poor. With an artificial pacemaker, life expectancy closely approaches that of the general population, although those with overt coronary heart disease or with heart failure have a less positive outlook. Pacemaker implantation should be considered in asymptomatic patients with complete AV block, particularly when the ventricular rate is 40 beats per minute or less, on purely prognostic grounds (4).

CONGENITAL HEART BLOCK

Congenital heart block, namely complete AV block that is discovered as a neonate or child and is not caused by acquired disease, is widely regarded as benign. However, some patients do develop symptoms or die suddenly. If heart block has caused symptoms, then pacing is indicated. In young asymptomatic patients, the risks of not implanting a pacemaker have to be weighed against the possibility of complications associated with several decades of pacing. There are several documented risk factors indicating a need for a pacemaker, such as daytime ventricular rate of less than 50 beats per minute, broad QRS complexes, pauses of more than 3.0 seconds, frequent ventricular ectopic beats and poor response of the heart rate to exercise. Unpaced patients should undergo ambulatory and exercise electrocardiography at regular intervals (4).

TACHYCARDIA

Atrial tachycardia is a supraventricular tachycardia, which means that the impulse driving the rapid rhythm originates above the ventricles, namely from within the atria, but not from the sinus node (see Figure 11.7). Atrial tachycardia has an atrial rate of from 150 to 250 beats per minute. This rapid rate shortens the diastole, resulting in a loss of atrial kick (that extra 30% of blood flow pushed into the ventricles by atrial contraction) (3). The increased ventricular rate from the atrial tachycardia results in a decrease in the time allowed for the ventricles to fill, an increase in myocardial oxygen consumption and a decrease in oxygen supply. Angina, heart failure, ischaemic myocardial changes and even a MI may result. A patient may complain of palpitations, blurred vision, syncope and hypotension (3).

Implantation of anti-tachycardia pacemakers is rarely needed nowadays, as radio-frequency ablation offers definitive treatment for supraventricular (SVT) arrhythmias. However, anti-tachycardia pacing is still useful in certain situations, such as:

- as part of tiered therapy with an implantable cardioverter defibrillator (ICD) in the management of VT;
- as an emergency in the catheter laboratory (cath lab) when SVT or VT may occur during cardiac catheterisation;
- in the coronary care unit or the intensive care unit, where drug therapy has failed or is inappropriate;
- very occasionally in patients with permanent pacemakers by programming the rate up and the AV delay down; permanent overdrive pacing may help to prevent VT (20).

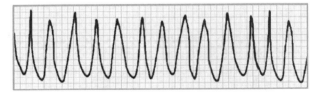

Figure 11.7. ECG strip showing ventricular tachycardia.

MANAGEMENT OF CHRONIC HEART FAILURE

Biventricular pacing – also known as cardiac resynchronisation therapy – has been successful in reducing symptoms and improving the quality of life in patients with advanced heart failure (3). In many patients with severe heart failure, the electrical impulse that induces ventricular contraction is delayed as it spreads across the myocardium. As a consequence, the regions of the ventricle activated earliest may be relaxing by the time the later regions start to contract (12). Typically, the interventricular septum contracts earlier than the delayed contraction of the lateral wall of the left ventricle. If opposing ventricular walls fail to contract together, a sizeable portion of blood is shifted around the left ventricle and is not ejected into circulation, thereby reducing cardiac output (8).

Unlike other pacemakers, a biventricular pacemaker can have three leads instead of two (see Figure 11.8). The leads in the right atrium and right ventricle are inserted in the same manner as that for an ordinary dual-chamber pacemaker (12). The coronary sinus is used for access to place a lead in the lateral wall of the left ventricle. As this lead is not anchored in place, it has a risk of lead displacement (3). Simultaneous pacing at the two ventricles results in a narrowing of QRS width and an improvement in cardiac output (12). Biventricular pacing improves left-ventricular remodelling and diastolic function and reduces sympathetic stimulation. As a result, in many patients, the progression of heart failure is slowed and their quality of life improved (3).

Unfortunately, not all patients with heart failure will benefit from biventricular pacing. Candidates should have both systolic heart failure and ventricular dyssynchrony, with these characteristics:

- symptomatic heart failure despite maximal medical therapy;
- moderate to severe heart failure (New York Association Class III or IV);

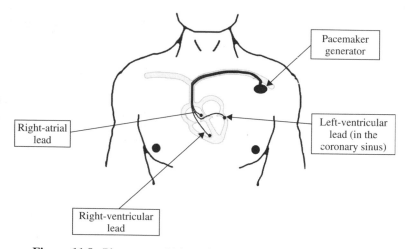

Figure 11.8. Placement of biventricular pacemaker on the left side.

- QRS complex of more than 0.13 seconds or 120 ms;
- evidence of incoordinate left-ventricular contraction on echocardiography (12).

PACEMAKER CODES

With the increasing complexity of permanent pacemakers, codes have been developed to enable healthcare staff to identify the capabilities of individual devices. Pacemaker function is described by a code established by the North American Society of the Pacing and Electrophysiology Group (NASPE) and the British Pacing and Electrophysiology Group (BPEG). The code, known as the NASPE/BPEG generic code, has undergone several revisions as pacemakers have acquired more functions (9).

The pacer mode is identified by at least three letters signifying (in order): (a) the chamber paced; (b) the chamber sensed; and (c) the response to sensed events. Additional letters may be appended to signify (d) programmability or rate modulation and (e) anti-tachycardia function (2) (see Table 11.1).

The first character identifies the chamber or chambers that are paced: A for atrium; V for ventricle; and D for dual if both atrium and ventricle can be stimulated (4).

The second character indicates the chamber or chambers in which intrinsic cardiac activity is sensed: in addition to the use of A, V and D, O indicates that the pacemaker is insensitive to the heart's intrinsic activity (4).

The third character denotes the pacemaker's response to the sensed information. The letter I means that the pacemaker is *inhibited* from firing in response to a

Table 11.1. Pacemaker codes

Code letter position	1st	2nd	3rd	4th	5th
Category	*Chamber(s) paced*	*Chamber(s) sensed*	*Mode of pacemaker response*	*Programmable functions*	*Tachyarrhythmia functions*
Letters used	V – ventricle A – atrium D – dual O – none	V – ventricle A – atrium D – dual O – none	I – inhibited T – triggered D – dual O – none	P – able to program simple functions M – able to program multi-programmable parameters C – has communicating functions such as telemetry R – rate responsiveness O – has none of the above functions	P – pacing ability S – shock D – dual ability to shock and pace

sensed intrinsic beat. For example, if the pacemaker is set at a rate of 70, the pacemaker will not fire if the patient's own heart rate is faster than 70 beats per minute. The pacemaker will fire only if the patient's intrinsic rate drops below the paced rate. The letter T in the third position indicates that the pacemaker will trigger a pacing impulse in response to a sensed intrinsic beat. For example, if a patient has a sinus rhythm but a complete AV block, their own intrinsic heartbeat will depolarise the atria but not the ventricles. The pacemaker is able to sense the atria's depolarising and will *trigger* the ventricles to depolarise appropriately. The letter D in this position designates a *dual* response in that it can inhibit pacing output when required and trigger pacing after sensing an event. The letter O indicates that the pacemaker does not respond to sensed intrinsic activity. This would be used in an asynchronous pacemaker (15).

A fourth character describes the pacemaker's programmability; this letter tells whether an external programming device can modify the pacemaker. The character R in the fourth position stands for 'rate responsiveness'. This feature can sense the need for increasing the heart rate, during periods of exercise, for example, and respond appropriately (3).

A programmable pacemaker can be non-invasively adjusted in one or more of its functions by radio-frequency signals emitted from an external programming device. Programmability enables achievement of optimal pacemaker function for the individual patient and can also be used in the diagnosis and treatment of certain pacemaker complications, thereby potentially reducing the need for pacemaker re-operation (4).

The fifth character only relates to anti-tachycardia pacemakers: O refers to none; P refers to pacing ability (the pacemaker initiates rapid bursts to pace the heart rate above its intrinsic rate to override the source of the tachycardia); S refers to shock (an implantable cardioverter–defibrillator identifies VT and delivers a shock to stop the arrhythmia); and D refers to dual ability to shock and pace (3).

EVALUATING PACEMAKERS

Using the NASPE/BPEG code to identify the type of pacemaker that the patient has can help to evaluate whether the pacemaker is functioning correctly when looking at a rhythm strip or electrocardiogram (ECG) (10). Pacing impulses are visible on ECG tracings. They are referred to as pacing spikes and are normally seen just before depolarisation of the cardiac muscle (3). Depending on the position of the electrode, the spike appears in different locations on the wave-form.

With an AAIR, the electrode is positioned in the atria only. Therefore, a pacing spike will be followed by a *P* wave and the patient's baseline QRS complex and *T* wave. The *P* waves may look different from the patient's normal *P* waves (3).

With a VVIR, the electrode is positioned in the ventricle only. The pacing spike will be followed by a wide QRS complex and *T* wave. There should be no equivalent of PR gap on the ECG, as the pacing wire is in direct contact with the myocardial tissue. The QRST complexes with pacing are often very large and wide, but they should be consistent in shape (10).

With a DDDR, there is an electrode positioned in the atria and the ventricle. The first spike is followed by a *P* wave, then a spike and then a wide QRS complex (3).

TYPES OF PERMANENT PACEMAKER

Whilst the electrical stimuli produced by a pacemaker are usually delivered to the heart by transvenous leads, less common methods such as transoesophageal or epicardial can be used when necessary:

- *Transoesophageal pacing* is more suitable for atrial pacing. A special high-output pacemaker (20 mA) is needed. An advantage is that it avoids requiring vascular access because the oesophagus acts as a conduit to the heart and is useful in the presence of coagulation abnormalities, venous access difficulties or terminating arrhythmias in which treatment with drugs is not suitable, such as pregnancy (10).
- The *epicardial* approach ensures excellent electrode stability but requires open-chest surgery. The electrodes are patches that are sewn to the outer layer of the heart and the pacemaker box is usually positioned under the skin of the abdomen. Epicardial systems tend to be less reliable in the long term. Wire displacement and fracture may occur due to kinking and vigorous movement; however, it is used in:
  - recurrent failure of endocardial systems due to infections, exit block, etc.;
  - small children in whom rapid growth makes transvenous pacing difficult;
  - heart block developing during cardiac surgery;
  - tricuspid mechanical valve prosthesis (20).

INSERTION OF A PERMANENT PACEMAKER

As about 95% of pacemakers are implanted *transvenously* and the pulse generator is implanted in a subcutaneous or sub-muscular pocket in the pectoral region below the clavicle (4), this will be the method described here. Venous access can be afforded by the subclavian, cephalic or axillary vein (2).

Single-chamber pacemakers have only one lead, connected to the heart in either the right atrium or the right ventricle. Dual-chamber pacemakers have a lead connected to the right atria and the right ventricle (24). Biventricular pacemakers have a third lead, placed against the left ventricle via the coronary sinus. However, this electrode is not anchored in place, which increases its risk of lead displacement (3). The technique of implanting a dual-chamber pacemaker is described here, as all pacemaker implants follow the same technique. The implant of a single-chamber device is slightly shorter, as it does not involve the placement of the second lead (2), whilst the biventricular implant will be longer for placing the more technically difficult left ventricular lead.

The majority of pacemakers are inserted around the left pectoral muscle, as it is easier for lead introduction and positioning. In addition, right-handed patients prefer the left side. However, the right side can also be used if the left is inaccessible or preferable (e.g. very active left-handed golfers or tennis players, etc.) (2).

WHAT A PATIENT CAN EXPECT WHEN UNDERGOING A PERMANENT PACEMAKER INSERTION

PRIOR TO THE PROCEDURE

Prior to admission, in order to minimise bleeding complications, patients should be advised to discontinue aspirin 1 week before the procedure, if possible (2). If a patient is on anticoagulation therapy such as warfarin, they should be advised to stop taking it at least 4 days before the procedure. The international normalised ratio (INR) should then be checked on the day of the procedure, to ensure that it is 1.5 or less (2). After pacemaker implantation, heparin use tends to be avoided if possible, as it may cause a haematoma around the pacemaker. Warfarin should be restarted on the evening of the implant rather than continuing with heparin (20).

On the patient's admission to the ward, the nurse will complete the patient's biographical details, taking note of past medical history and allergies. Any problems identified should be discussed with the medical staff. For example, if the patient had developed an infection such as a chest infection, this should be treated before implanting the pacemaker (2). Nursing staff will record the baseline observations, such as weight, height, pulse, blood pressure, temperature and blood glucose if the patient is diabetic (25). If necessary, chest hairs should be shaved; then the patient will be asked to change into a surgical gown (25).

A peripheral intravenous cannula should be inserted prior to the procedure, preferably into the side to be proceeded on, as an injection of radiographic contrast dye may be required during the procedure (2).

To reduce the risk of infection, prophylactic antibiotics should be administered (2). If pre-medication, such as diazepam, is prescribed to reduce anxiety, this should be administered 45–70 minutes before the procedure. The informed consent should be signed before administering it, as it may make the patient sleepy (14).

As the pacemaker is inserted under local anaesthetic, patients do not have to fast prior to the procedure; they may have a light meal up to 2 hours beforehand (19).

DURING THE PROCEDURE

Patients should be informed that inserting a pacemaker may take 1–2 hours (23). Once the patient has been positioned on the table, cardiac monitoring leads will be attached to their torso. As meticulous sterile technique should be exercised throughout the procedure, they will feel the nursing staff clean the implant area with an iodine/antiseptic solution. Then, the area will be draped with sterile towels (2).

Once the patient is prepared, a local anaesthetic (1% lignocaine) is liberally inserted into the region to be incised. Where necessary, judicious use of an intravenous benzodiazepine (e.g. midazolam) and/or a narcotic (e.g. fentanyl) can be administered, as it reduces both patient anxiety and discomfort. The drugs should be short-acting to minimise the risk of severe respiratory depression (2). Once the area is anaesthetised, an incision is made through the skin. After further local anaesthesia, a subcutaneous or sub-muscular pocket is made with blunt and sharp dissection; then, depending on the cardiologist's preference, the wound may be irrigated liberally with antibiotic solution (2).

A variety of veins are available for gaining venous access. The cephalic vein cut-down approach is preferred, as venous access is achieved under direct visualisation and there is no risk of pneumothorax. In addition, some believe that there is a lower incidence of lead fraction due to crushing at the junction between the first rib and the clavicle (2). Alternatively, the axillary vein or subclavian vein can be used (2). The subclavian approach is now widely used and is especially useful if more than one lead is to be inserted. As the puncture of the subclavian vein is easier if the vein is distended, patients should be informed that the table may be tilted so that they will be in a slightly head-down position or, alternatively, that their legs may be raised (4). Since the subclavian puncture is performed without direct visualisation of the vein, there is a risk of pneumothorax and subclavian artery puncture (2).

Once venous access has been achieved, a guidewire is then inserted. This is used to introduce the venous sheath into the vein. The venous sheath itself is used to introduce the longer and softer pacemaker lead into the vein. The venous sheath is of the 'peel-away' type, to allow its removal after the lead has been inserted. When the lead is being introduced, the patient may be instructed to stop breathing (without taking a deep breath first) in order to minimise the risk of an air embolism (2).

The ventricular lead is first advanced to the right atrium. Pacemaker leads are intentionally designed to be flexible; this lack of axial stiffness helps to prevent cardiac perforation by the leads. However, such flexible leads are not easily manipulated, and the use of a stiffening wire stylet is required. Using this stylet, the ventricle lead is passed through the tricuspid valve and into the right ventricle towards the apex. The sheath is then withdrawn from the vein and removed (retaining the guidewire if another lead is to be placed) (2).

As ventricular ectopy is common during lead manipulation, patients should be warned that they may feel that their heart is beating faster whilst the lead is being manoeuvred; however, the ventricular ectopy almost always stops when the lead position is stable (2). Once a good lead position is established by x-ray, the electrode is then placed into the myocardium followed by careful withdrawal of the stylet (2).

Sensing of the R waves and pacing threshold are then checked for acceptable function. Inadequate sensing or pacing, despite a good anatomic site, suggests an injured area of myocardium, though the integrity of the lead, the testing equipment and all connections must be confirmed before repositioning (2). In addition, an ECG should be examined (especially lead V1) during pacing to ensure the presence of a left bundle branch block pattern. Right bundle branch block suggests pacing from the left ventricle, which may occur if the lead crossed the atrial or ventricular septum, if the lead is inadvertently placed in one of the cardiac veins via the coronary sinus or if the lead has perforated the heart and pacing is occurring from the left-ventricular epicardium (2).

After good ventricular lead placement is achieved, the atrial lead can be inserted. Using the retained wire as a guide, a second peel-away sheath is advanced into the vein. The atrial lead is then advanced and placed in the atrium. The right atrial appendage has been identified as being an ideal site for lead placement. Once the electrode is securely positioned, the electrogram is examined to ensure atrial sensing. The ventricular lead is also examined to ensure that it has not been displaced (2).

After satisfactory positions for both leads are found, the leads will be examined under fluoroscopy, and the patient will be asked to breathe in deeply and cough vigorously to ensure that the lead tips are not dislodged by these actions (2). Pacing at high output will be performed to ensure that there is no pacing of the diaphragm, particularly by the atrial lead, since the right phrenic nerve courses along the lateral right atrium (2).

Once a good position for both electrodes has been confirmed, they are anchored by stitching the leads in place, using strong non-absorbable sutures (2). Then, the pacemaker pulse generator is connected to the lead(s). The system is then implanted into the pocket, with the lead(s) coiled behind the generator to minimise the risk of damage to the leads in the event of re-incision. The pocket is then closed using two layers of an absorbable suture. The incision may be closed with adhesive tape (such as steri-strips) and then covered with a gauze dressing (2). Alternatively, depending on the cardiologist's preference, the incision may be sealed by a tissue adhesive, such as Dermabond, instead (18). In order to minimise haematoma formation in the incision site, some patients may have a drain inserted and/or have a pressure dressing applied (18).

POST-PROCEDURE CARE

After successful pacemaker implantation, the primary risk in the early post-procedure period is lead displacement. Therefore, patients are advised to remain on bed rest overnight and the arm adjacent to where the pacemaker is inserted may be put in a sling to restrict movement (2). Whilst the patient is on bed rest, they should be attached to a continuous cardiac monitor to ensure that the pacemaker is working normally. Four-hourly temperature, pulse and respiration should be recorded (10). If a drain has been inserted, this should be checked regularly and emptied when required. In order to reduce the risk of infection, the drain should be handled as little as possible, and an aseptic technique used when doing so (18).

Although complications are rare following a permanent pacemaker insertion, they do occur in 0.5% of cases and are often serious (10); therefore, nurses should observe for:

- signs of infection;
- surgical emphysema around the pacemaker insertion site; air enters the subcutaneous tissue and it feels crunchy under your fingertips;
- pectoral muscle twitching or hiccups that occur in synchrony with the pacemaker;
- cardiac tamponade; signs and symptoms include persistent hiccups, distant heart sounds, a drop in the strength of a pulse during inspiration, hypotension with a narrowed pulse pressure, cyanosis, distended jugular veins, decreased urine output, restlessness, complaints of a full chest;
- pneumothorax; signs and symptoms include shortness of breath, restlessness and hypoxia; mental status changes and arrhythmias may also occur; diminished breath sounds, usually on the apex of the lung on the side in which the pacemaker was implanted (3); a pneumothorax can normally be seen on a chest x-ray (15).

Anticoagulation should be withheld for several hours to minimise the risk of bleeding and haematoma in the pacemaker pocket (2). In suitable patients, warfarin should be restarted on the evening of the implantation rather than continuing with heparin (20).

As the pacemaker site may be bruised, swollen and tender, especially if a submuscular pocket was created, prescribed analgesia should be administered (23) with the prophylactic antibiotics (2).

The drain is usually removed the day after the procedure. As with all drains, it should be removed when the drainage has stopped. First, ensure that any vacuum or suction in the drain is released. Then, using an aseptic technique, the retaining suture should be cut and removed. Using gentle pressure, the drain should be withdrawn. If it does not come out easily, inform the medical staff, as it may have become entangled with the pacemaker or the wires. Once removed, a small absorbent dressing should be applied to the drain site and observed for excessive amounts of leakage until healing has occurred (18).

The incision site should be inspected for signs of bleeding or infection and the patient informed about how to care for it. Although wounds closed with steri-strips or Dermabond do not normally need an absorbent dressing to cover them, considering where the site is, some patients prefer one to prevent their clothing from irritating the wound (especially ladies wearing bras or men wearing braces).

When the subclavian vein is used, a portable chest x-ray should be taken on the ward, on the same day as the procedure, to exclude a pneumothorax as well as to verify lead position. No matter which vein is used for access, it is recommended that a posterior–anterior and lateral chest x-ray should be taken the day after the procedure to examine the stability of lead placement (2).

Before discharge, the pacemaker is interrogated to ensure that no marked changes in lead impedance, pacing threshold or sensing have occurred. Such changes raise the possibility of lead displacement (2). Once it has been established that the leads have not been displaced, the patient is allowed to mobilise.

Patients with implanted pacemakers should regularly attend a follow-up clinic. The purposes are: to check that the pacemaker is working satisfactorily; to ensure that there are no pacing complications; to detect impending battery depletion so that generator replacement can be carried out before the patient is at risk; and to maintain a record of patients' locations should a recall of a particular generator or lead be necessary (4). The pacemaker battery lasts about 5–10 years, depending on its usage. The battery usually provides several months' warning indicating that it needs replacing (24).

The Pacemaker Clinic visits following the first visit for a wound check can be timed to follow the post-implantation threshold rise. For example, a 1-month visit would be near the peak of the threshold rise. Another visit at 3 months would coincide with the threshold's reaching the chronic state. The output of the pacing stimulus can then be reduced (maintaining an adequate safety margin) to maximise battery life. Routine follow-up should always include a history of any new symptoms as well as an examination of the pocket site for erythema, oedema, tenderness or threatened erosion (2).

Patients with permanent pacemakers are often discharged the following day and any non-dissolvable sutures (if used) can be taken out 5 days later at the family doctor's surgery. Future pacemaker checks can be carried out on an out-patient basis. Finally, patients should be given comprehensive discharge advice geared to their intellectual capacity and age (10).

DISCHARGE ADVICE

Upon discharge, patients should be advised:

1. Keep the incision site dry; wait until the third day before having a shower (23).
2. Avoid raising the arm adjacent to the incision site for the first week; shirts or cardigans that button at the front are easier to put on (23).
3. For 1–2 months, do not lift, push or pull anything that weighs more than 5 pounds (2.3 kg), including groceries and children (23).

4. For 1–2 months, avoid arm exercises or activities, like sweeping, that require repeated movement of the arm (23).

5. Do not put pressure on the incision site, such as by wearing braces or tight clothes, until the incision has healed (23).

6. People with pacemakers are still legally required to wear seatbelts, but, until the incision has healed, they may find it more comfortable to wear it across the shoulder opposite the incision site.

7. Tell your other healthcare professionals, such as your dentist, that you have had a pacemaker inserted (23).

8. Vigorous contact sports, such as rugby, boxing or judo, should be avoided in order to avoid injury to the pacemaker (20).

9. A pacemaker may set off metal detectors or some anti-theft devices, so people with pacemakers should carry their pacemaker ID card to show authorities, if required (23).

10. Do not drive until advised to by the cardiologist (23). The DVLA (2006) recommends no driving for 1 week after the procedure for group 1 drivers. People who drive large lorries and buses fall into group 2 and are not allowed to drive for 6 weeks after a pacemaker insertion (7).

11. Inform your cardiologist if there:
    • is any recurrence of your previous symptoms (23);
    • is any sign of infection in the incision site, such as swelling, fluid, pain, redness (or other unusual colour at the pacemaker site), chills or a temperature of 38 °C or higher (23);
    • are hiccups that last more than 15 minutes (23).

When providing the discharge advice, the opportunity should be used to disabuse patients and their families/carers about common misconceptions about pacemakers arising from popular notions or outdated information (see Chapter 13).

COMPLICATIONS

The risks associated with transvenous implantation of a permanent pacemaker are low. Nonetheless, complications do occur, and the patient should be apprised of the risk in the informed-consent process before the procedure. Some complications present later and Table 11.2 lists potential complications that may occur following a pacemaker implantation (2). Nursing staff should be aware of all the potential complications, especially the early ones, so that they know what to look for post procedure. These are discussed in more detail in Chapter 13.

CARE PLANS

PROBLEM/NEED

Patient is to have a permanent pacemaker inserted.

Table 11.2. Complications of transvenous pacemaker or ICD implantation

Early complications	Late complications
Infection	Lead dislodgment
Bleeding	Erosion of skin over pocket
Pneumothorax/hemothorax	Pain
Air embolism	Infection
Arterial cannulation	Lead fracture
Perforation of heart/tamponade	Lead insulation failure
Atrial fibrillation	Infection
Heart block induced by contact	Migration of pulse generator
with conduction system	Twisting and fracture of leads due to
Deep vein thrombosis	manipulation of generator – twiddlers
Lead damage fracture	syndrome
Lead dislodgment	
Ventricular tachycardia	
Pocket haematoma	
Incorrect connection of leads to	
pulse generator	

Source: Baim and Grossman (2000) *Cardiac Catheterisation, Angiography and Intervention 6E*. Reproduced by permission of Lippincott, Williams and Wilkins, London.

PRE-PROCEDURE CARE PLAN FOR PATIENTS UNDERGOING A PERMANENT PACEMAKER IMPLANTATION

Goal/aim of care

Patient to be prepared for permanent pacemaker insertion, ensuring pre, peri and post-procedure safety.

Action	Rationale
Obtain a brief history and check that biographical details and next of kin are correct	Checking the patient's biographical details and next of kin ensures that medical records are up-to-date and, in the event of an emergency, the correct person is contacted. Record keeping is a fundamental part of nursing care, ensuring high standards of clinical care, and improving communication and dissemination of information (16)
Explain the procedure to the patient and significant others, to alleviate anxieties	The period before any procedure may cause extreme anxiety in some patients. Discussion and reassurance may help to relieve some of these feelings (11)
Check whether the patient is allergic to any food, drugs or other substances. Inform the doctor if the patient is allergic to	Patients with a history of allergy to iodine-containing substances, such as seafood or contrast agents, should be given an antihistamine and steroids

Action	Rationale
any potential drugs used in the procedure	before the procedure (25). In addition to this, a non-ionic contrast dye may be used for the procedure (5)
Warfarin should be stopped at least 48 hours prior to the procedure	Warfarin should be withheld for at least 48 hours prior to the procedure to ensure an INR of less than 1.5. Patients at high risk for thromboembolism should be admitted for heparinisation while the effects of oral anticoagulation wane (5)
Ideally, the INR should be less than 1.5 (inform the cardiologist if it is higher)	Warfarin interferes with blood coagulation by blocking the effect of vitamin K. It has a long-acting half-life of 36–42 hours. The anticoagulation effect is described in a measurement of the INR. Therefore, any INR measurement of more than 1.5 increases the patient's risk of bleeding uncontrollably during and/or after the procedure (6)
Check that the patient has stopped their aspirin for at least 1 week prior to the procedure, when appropriate	To minimise bleeding during the procedure (2)
Obtain baseline blood pressure, pulse, temperature, respiration rate and blood glucose	In order to provide a baseline for comparison after the pacemaker has been inserted (10)
Record the patient's height and weight	The amount of some of the drugs prescribed during the procedure may be calculated on the patient's body weight (2; 14)
Cannulate the patient, preferably on the same side as the pacemaker is to be inserted	To provide intravenous access to administer prescribed drugs (10). Radio-opaque contrast may be used to visualise a vein during the procedure (2)
Ensure that identification and allergy bands are correct, legible and secure	To ensure correct identification and prevent possible problems (25)

Action	Rationale
Ensure that the skin is shaved where they intend to insert the pacemaker	Body hair is removed in order to reduce infection risk (25)
Patients may wear dentures, glasses and hearing aids during the procedure	Patients are better able to communicate when dentures and hearing aids are in place. Glasses allow the patient to view the procedure better and help to keep the patient oriented to the surroundings (25)
Encourage the patient to empty their bladder prior to taking the pre-medication/procedure	To help make them more comfortable (25)
Ensure that the informed consent has been signed	The procedure and its risks should be explained and the patient's questions should be answered before the procedure (2)
If the patient is a female of child-bearing age, she may be asked by the radiographer to sign a form indicating her pregnancy status	Pregnancy is a relative contraindicator in cardiac intervention procedures (13). However, as direct irradiation of the uterus can usually be avoided in procedures that involve structures above the diaphragm, fluoroscopic procedures on pregnant women may be justifiable in an emergency situation (2)

POST-PROCEDURE CARE PLAN

Goal/aim of care

The nursing care of patients following permanent pacemaker insertion is directed towards the prevention and detection of complications.

Action	Rationale
Attach the patient to a cardiac monitor and obtain blood pressure and pulse readings	The heart rhythm should be monitored after a pacemaker insertion to ensure that the pacemaker is pacing properly (2; 10)
Check blood pressure and temperature 4-hourly post procedure	In order to observe for any haemodynamic compromise (10)

Action	Rationale
If the patient is a diabetic, check their blood sugar on warding	To ensure that the patient is not hypoglycaemic, as they may have fasted for long periods prior to the procedure (25)
Encourage the patient to drink and provide them with something to eat	Patients are often tired, hungry and uncomfortable when they return from the laboratory. Patients should be encouraged to drink plenty in order to prevent hypotension (25)
Ensure that any intravenous pumps are running at the correct rate, and administer any drugs prescribed post procedure	It is the ward nurses' responsibility to ensure that the prescribed drugs, intravenous or oral, are administered correctly (17)
If a drain was inserted, regularly check and empty the drain	To minimise haematoma formation (18)
If the subclavian vein was utilised, obtain a portable chest x-ray on the ward	It is difficult to identify a pneumothorax or haemothorax on chest x-ray when the patient is lying down; therefore, the patient should have an upright chest x-ray when the subclavian vein is used (2)
Advise patients to take things slowly when they first mobilise	A patient may drop their blood pressure by simply standing up abruptly after prolonged bed rest (21)
Prior to discharge, re-dress the incision and look for signs of weeping, redness or inflammation	To check for signs of excessive bleeding or infection (2; 10)
Discharge home with both verbal and written advice	Discharge information should be given in both written and verbal forms, ensuring that patients understand this prior to leaving (10)
Any changes in medication should be discussed with the patient	When discharging a patient, it is the nurses' responsibility to inform the patient about the medication that they have been prescribed so that they will take it correctly at home (17)

BOX CHANGE

As the pacemaker batteries have a finite lifetime, it is necessary to change the pacemaker box. The procedure is simpler that the original implantation because the leads do not need to be replaced or moved, unless they have been damaged at the time of checking. In pacemaker-dependent patients and those at risk of profound bradycardia, a temporary transvenous pacemaker will be required first (2).

Changing a pacemaker box is similar to having a pacemaker implanted, in that it is performed under sterile conditions in the cath lab. Local anaesthesia is injected into the incision site that will provide access to the original pacemaker. This will probably be surrounded by fibrous tissue, so this will have to be incised to loosen the pacemaker. Once free, the pacemaker will be disconnected from its leads. At this stage, all the leads will be checked to ensure that they are still working. Then, the new pacemaker is attached to the existing leads. Depending on the cardiologist's preference, before implanting the pacemaker, the pocket is irrigated with an antibiotic solution to minimise the risk of infection. Then, the wound is closed in a similar manner as that for a pacemaker (2).

Post-procedure wound care, including prophylactic antibiotic therapy, is similar to post-procedure care of the original implant. However, an overnight stay in hospital and post-procedure x-rays are unnecessary in uncomplicated cases, since the leads are chronic and the risk of dislodgment is low (2).

REFERENCES

1. Al-Obaidi, M., Siva, A. and Noble, M. (2004) 'Crash Course Cardiology', 2nd edn, London, Mosby.
2. Baim, D. S. and Grossman, W. (2000) 'Grossman's Cardiac Catheterisation: Angiography and Intervention', 6th edn, London, Lippincott Williams & Wilkins.
3. Beverage, D., Haworth, K., Labus, D., Mayer, B. and Munson, S. (2005) ECG Interpretation Made Incredibly Easy, London, Lippincott Williams & Wilkins.
4. Bennett, D. H. (2002) Cardiac Arrhythmias: Practical Notes on Interpretation and Treatment, London, Arnold.
5. Braunwald, E., Zipes, D. and Libby, P. (2001) Heart Disease: A Textbook of Cardiovascular Medicine, 6th edn, Philadelphia, PA, W.B. Saunders Co.
6. Blann, A., Landray, M. and Lip, G. (2002) 'An overview of antithrombotic therapy', British Medical Journal, 325: 762–5.
7. DVLA (2006) For Medical Practitioners: At a Glance Guide to the Current Medical Standards for Fitness to Drive, February, available online at www.DVLA.gov.uk.
8. Frodsham, R. (2005) 'Cardiac resynchronisation therapy for patients with heart failure', Nursing Standard, 19(45): 46–50.
9. Geiter, H. (2004) 'Getting back to basics with permanent pacemakers: Part 1', Nursing, 34(10): 32cc1–4.
10. Hubbard, J. (2003) 'An overview of permanent and temporary cardiac pacemakers', Nursing Times, 99(36): 26–7.
11. Hughes, S. (2002) 'The effects of pre-operative information', Nursing Standard, 16: 28, 33–7.

12. Julian, D. G., Cowan, J. C. and McLenachan, J. M. (2005) *'Cardiology'*, 8th edn, London, Elsevier Saunders.
13. Kern, M. (2003) *The Cardiac Catheterisation Handbook*, 4th edn, London, Mosby.
14. Lemone, P. and Burke, K. (2004) *Medical/Surgical Nursing: Critical Thinking in Client Care*, 3rd edn, Upper Saddle River, NJ, Prentice Hall.
15. Morton, P., Fontaine, D., Hudak, C. and Gallo, B. (2005) *Critical Care Nursing: A Holistic Approach*, 8th edn, Philadelphia, PA, Lippincott Williams and Wilkins.
16. Nursing Midwifery Council (2002a) *Guidelines for Records and Record Keeping*, London, Nursing and Midwifery Council, April.
17. Nursing Midwifery Council (2002b) *Guidelines for the Administration of Medicines*, London, Nursing and Midwifery Council.
18. Pudner, R. (2000) *Nursing the Surgical Patient*, London, Bailliere Tindall.
19. Soreide, E., Eriksson, L. I., Hirlekar, G., Eriksson, H., Henneberg, W., Sandin, R. and Raeder, J. (Task Force on Scandinavian Pre-operative Fasting Guidelines, Clinical Practice Committee Scandinavian Society of Anaesthesiology and Intensive Care Medicine) (2005) 'Pre-operative fasting guidelines: An update', *Acta Anaesthesiologica Scandinavica*, **49**: 1041–7.
20. Swanton, R. H. (2003) *Cardiology*, 5th edn, Malden, MA, Blackwell Publishing.
21. Topol, E. J. (1999) *Textbook of Interventional Cardiology*, 3rd edn, London, W.B. Saunders Co.
22. Tortora, G. J. and Derrickson, B. (2006) *Principles of Anatomy and Physiology*, 8th edn, Chichester, John Wiley and Sons Inc.
23. Toth, P. and Knect, J. (2004) 'Pacemakers', *Nursing*, **34**(1): 46–7.
24. Wood, M. A. and Ellenbogen, K. A. (2002) 'Cardiac pacemakers from the patient's perspective', *Circulation*, **105**: 1136–8.
25. Woods, S., Froelicher, E. and Motzer, S. (2000) *Cardiac Nursing*, 4th edn, Philadelphia, PA, Lippincott Williams & Wilkins.

12 Implantable Cardioverter Defibrillators

SUDDEN CARDIAC DEATH

An electrical malfunction of the heart can lead to a loss of cardiac output and effective pulse from which, if it remains untreated, the patient will die. This is termed as 'sudden cardiac death' (SCD) and occurs in approximately 50,000–70,000 people throughout the United Kingdom each year. The largest proportion of deaths from coronary heart disease is attributed to an SCD event (21). The use of the term 'sudden cardiac death' is potentially misleading, as it implies that death has occurred; however, such events are survivable (19). NICE (2006) estimates that fewer than 5% of people survive the initial 'out-of-hospital' event (21).

NICE (2006) estimate that about 80% of SCD events are caused by ventricular tachyarrhythmia, such as ventricular tachycardia (VT) and/or ventricular fibrillation (VF). The remaining 20% consists of a number of conditions, including cardiomyopathy (10–15%), other structural heart defects (less than 5%) and bradycardia (21). Ventricular tachycardia is defined as three or more consecutive ventricular beats occurring at a rate of more than 120 beats per minute (1) (see Figure 12.1). This is an extremely unstable rhythm, which can occur in short, paroxysmal bursts lasting less than 30 seconds, resulting in few or no symptoms. Some patients can maintain their pulse with a longer period of VT; however, because of the reduced ventricular filling time, cardiac output will fall and the patient's condition can quickly deteriorate into VF and death (4). Ventricular fibrillation is an irregular rapid depolarisation of the ventricles (see Figure 12.2) so that there is no organised contraction, the ventricles quiver rather than contract, and therefore the patient will have no pulse. If it remains untreated, this rapidly leads to death (1).

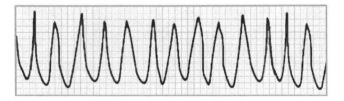

Figure 12.1. ECG strip of ventricular tachycardia.

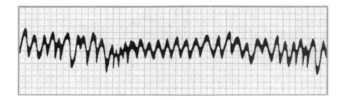

Figure 12.2. ECG strip of ventricular fibrillation.

Even with treatment of the underlying cause of the VT/VF, about 10–15% of the survivors of an SCD event are at increased risk of a second event. If this second SCD event is not treated promptly, it is usually fatal (21). As defibrillation is the most effective treatment for VT and VF, survivors of an SCD event may be offered an implantable cardioverter defibrillator (ICD) (4).

WHAT IS AN IMPLANTABLE CARDIOVERTER DEFIBRILLATOR?

An ICD is an electronic device implanted in the body to provide continuous monitoring of the heart for bradycardia, VT and VF. The device then administers either paced beats or shocks to treat the dangerous arrhythmia. In general, ICDs are indicated for patients for whom drug therapy, surgery or radio-frequency ablation has failed to prevent the arrhythmia (4).

ICDs are similar to a pacemaker, but are slightly larger, to accommodate their increased functions. They are usually implanted in a similar manner – the box is implanted in a subcutaneous or sub-muscular pocket in the left pectoral region below the clavicle and the leads are inserted intravenously into the atrium and ventricle (6) (see Figure 12.3).

Modern ICDs can provide tiered therapy – the term used to describe different levels of therapy to terminate a dysrhythmia. The first tier of therapy is usually *anti-tachycardia pacing*, which involves the use of rapid overdrive pacing to 'overcome' and 'recapture' the heart rhythm (10). If anti-tachycardia pacing is not successful, the second tier of therapy is initiated by the device. With the second tier, a low-energy synchronised *cardioversion* is delivered. This is when a low or high-energy shock (up to 35 joules) is timed to the *R* wave to terminate VT and return the heart to its normal rhythm (4). Some devices allow multiple attempts at cardioversion. If cardioversion is not successful, the third tier of therapy – *defibrillation* – is used. The energy delivered for defibrillation can be programmed to a maximum of 35 joules, again depending on the model and the capacity of the device. The number of defibrillation attempts varies with each device, but six attempts is usually the maximum. If the patient is successfully converted to a life-compatible rhythm, but the heart rate is slow, ventricular *demand pacing* is initiated. This fourth tier of therapy is usually intended for

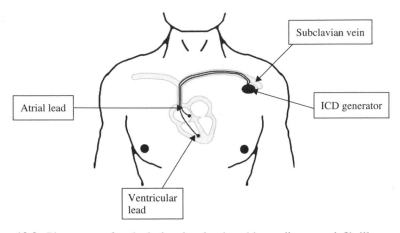

Figure 12.3. Placement of a dual chamber implantable cardioverter defibrillator on the left side.

brief periods of pacing until normal rhythm resumes (20). The advantage of the tiered therapy is that it allows the ICD to meet individualised patient electrophysiological needs. In some cases, the tiered therapy may reduce and even avoid the need for an internal defibrillating shock (10).

In addition to tiered therapy, modern ICDs offer many programmable features. Bradycardia pacing therapies with dual chamber defibrillators are a common feature of current ICDs. In addition, the availability of an atrial sensing lead allows for a more specific supraventricular tachycardia (SVT) discrimination algorithm. Some devices also have separate tiers of therapy for atrial tachycardias and atrial fibrillation/flutter. All of the current devices are 'noncommitted', meaning that therapy is aborted if the tachycardia terminates, even while the ICD is charging up. Therefore, patients with non-sustained VT need not suffer the discomfort of an inappropriate shock (20).

An ICD also stores information about the heart's activity before, during and after an arrhythmia, along with tracking which treatment was delivered and the outcome of that treatment. Many devices also store electrograms (electrical tracings similar to electrocardiograms (ECGs)). With an interrogation device, a doctor/technician or nurse with specialised training can retrieve this information to evaluate ICD function and battery status and to adjust ICD system settings (4).

WHO NEEDS AN IMPLANTABLE CARDIOVERTER DEFIBRILLATOR?

Implantable cardioverter defibrillators are recommended for people who are considered to be at high risk of SCD. These patients fall into two categories: secondary prevention and primary prevention (17). Secondary prevention of

SCD is defined as the prevention of an *additional life-threatening* event in survivors of sudden cardiac events or in patients with recurrent unstable cardiac rhythms, whilst primary prevention of SCD is defined as prevention of a *first life-threatening arrhythmic event* (21). This is usually targeted at known high-risk patients such as those with coronary artery disease and left ventricular dysfunction (10).

The NICE (2006) guidelines recommend that patients who fall into the following categories should have an ICD:

1. **Secondary prevention,** that is, for patients who present, in the absence of treatable cause, with one of the following:
   - Having survived a cardiac arrest due to either VT or VF
   - Spontaneous sustained VT causing syncope or significant haemodynamic compromise
   - Sustained VT without syncope or cardiac arrest, and who have an associated reduction in ejection fraction (LVEF of less than 35%) (no worse than class III of the New York Heart Association functional classification of heart failure) (21).
2. **Primary prevention,** that is, for patients who have a history of previous (more than 4 weeks) myocardial infarction and:
   Either
   - Left ventricular dysfunction with an LVEF of less that 35% (no worse than class III of the New York heart association functional classification of heart failure) **and**
   - Non-sustained VT on Holter monitoring **and**
   - Inducible VT on electrophysiological testing

   Or
   - Left ventricular dysfunction with an LVEF of less than 30% (no worse than class III of the New York Heart Association functional classification of heart failure) **and**
   - QRS duration of equal to or more than 120 milliseconds

   - A familial cardiac condition with a high risk of sudden death, including long QT syndrome, hypertrophic cardiomyopathy, Brugada syndrome, or arrhythmogenic right ventricular dysplasia (AVRD), or have undergone surgical repair of congenital heart disease (21).

The ejection fraction in patients with heart failure is reduced because the ventricles are not contracting in a synchronised manner. Recent studies have shown that pacing both right and left ventricles simultaneously improves the ejection fraction and cardiac output (17). This has been referred to as cardiac resynchronisation therapy (CRT), ventricular resynchronisation therapy (VRT) and biventricular pacing. As about 50% of patients with heart failure die from progressive heart failure and the other 50% die suddenly as a result of ventricular arrhythmias, it is not surprising that CRT has been added to the ICD's arsenal of functions for suitable patients (17).

CARDIAC RESYNCHRONISATION THERAPY

In many patients with severe heart failure, the electrical impulse that induces ventricular contraction is delayed as it spreads across the myocardium. As a consequence, the regions of the ventricle activated earliest may be relaxing by the time the later regions start to contract (17). Typically, the interventricular septum contracts earlier than the lateral wall of the left ventricle. This abnormal interventricular conduction is referred to as ventricular dyssynchrony. If opposing ventricular walls fail to contract together, a sizeable portion of blood is shifted around the left ventricle and is not ejected into circulation, thereby reducing cardiac output (11).

For CRT, a pacing electrode is placed in the apex of the right ventricle, just like conventional pacing (17). The coronary sinus is used to position the tip of a pacing electrode in the epicardial vein on the lateral wall of the left ventricle (11). As the electrodes are in direct contact with the myocardium in the left ventricular wall, this reduces the time required for ventricular activation, thus improving the synchronisation of contracting both ventricles. This results in a narrowing of QRS width and an improvement in cardiac output (17). Unfortunately, because the left ventricular lead is not anchored in place, it is at increased risk of displacement (4).

Criteria of selection of patients likely to benefit most from resynchronisation pacing include:

- severe heart failure, New York Heart Association class III or IV;
- left bundle branch block;
- QRS width greater than 120 ms;
- evidence of incoordinate left ventricular contraction on echocardiography (17).

CONTRAINDICATIONS TO IMPLANTABLE CARDIOVERTER DEFIBRILLATOR

Implantable cardioverter defibrillator therapy or implantation is not recommended in:

- patients in whom VT/VF is due to a reversible cause, such as acute myocardial infarction or severe electrolyte abnormalities;
- patients with ongoing infections should have the infection assessed and treated prior to implanting an ICD;
- patients with LV dysfunction undergoing routine bypass graft surgery without inducible sustained VT;
- patients with Wolff–Parkinsons–White syndrome should undergo catheter ablation of their accessory bypass tracts instead of receiving ICD therapy;

- patients with incessant VTs that are resistant to drugs may not benefit from ICDs because the arrhythmias would constantly trigger shocks. Surgical or catheter ablation should be attempted instead of ICD implantation;
- patients with terminal illnesses and life expectancy of less than 6 months;
- severe psychiatric disorders that may be worsened with ICD therapy or, if patients are unable to have ICD follow-up, they should not have the device implanted (2).

PSYCHOLOGICAL IMPACT OF HAVING AN IMPLANTABLE CARDIOVERTER DEFIBRILLATOR/QUALITY OF LIFE

Although an ICD is a life-saving device, ICD recipients experience a myriad of physical, emotional and social adjustments (12). Spouses and family members of ICD patients can also manifest emotional reactions by showing hypervigilance and overprotecting the ICD patient (10). However, by providing good pre-implantation education and follow-up support, these problems can be reduced (26). Areas of need identified include preparation for the physical aspects of being fitted with an ICD, explanations regarding practical adaptations to their lifestyle (e.g. the enforced driving ban for 6 months in the United Kingdom) and preparation for possible psychological responses (30).

The following is an indication of some of the concerns that an ICD recipient or their family might express.

ANXIETY

Anxiety is the most common psychosocial concern seen in ICD recipients after implantation (26). Anxieties range from fear of death, loss of control, device malfunction and problems with overprotective family members. Anxiety may result in trouble sleeping and loss of concentration. Patients should be assured that anxiety and depression are common reactions, but it may take 6 months to a year to make the adjustment to having an ICD (35). Patients concerned that resuming activities that increase their heart rate, such as exercise or sexual activity, may set off the device, therefore, may avoid these activities (12). Patients, however, should be encouraged to resume these activities. They should be reassured that it may be possible to increase the device's tachycardia detection level, if necessary, to avoid unnecessary shocks (20).

LOSS OF INDEPENDENCE

Loss of independence also contributes towards anxiety. Fear of being alone and depending on other people for activities such as driving may also be stressful (26). As driving is an important aspect of maintaining independence, driving restrictions can cause feelings of isolation, anger and loss of autonomy (20).

Currently, in the United Kingdom, patients who have an ICD implanted for primary prevention but were asymptomatic are not allowed to drive for 1 month after ICD implantation. Patients who have had an ICD implanted for secondary prevention have to inform the DVLA and are not allowed to drive for at least 6 months (9). It should be explained to the patient and their family that it is the symptoms associated with a ventricular arrhythmia and not the ICD that makes driving potentially dangerous (20).

Feelings of loss of control can be addressed, if not overcome, by nurses' providing extensive education which involves both the patient and the family. Patients and family members should be encouraged to express their true feelings and concerns about imminent events (such as the ICD implant and its implications) and potential lifestyle changes (19).

SOCIO-ECONOMIC

As ICD recipients may still be working, especially those receiving it for secondary prevention, how the ICD impacts on the job may be a major concern for the patient. If the patient works in an environment in which there are high levels of electromagnetic interference (EMI), such as electrical smelting furnaces, radio-frequency transmitters such as radar, high-voltage systems, theft-prevention equipment and high-powered electromagnetic fields, they may have to give up their job (20). Electromagnetic interference is defined as 'highly-regular electrical potentials of low amplitude and high frequency'; unfortunately, when this interacts with an ICD, it can result in inappropriate ICD discharges, rhythm-sensing problems and, occasionally, inhibition of cardiac pacing (35). Experts feel that sources of EMI must be in close proximity (within 6 inches/15 cm) to the patient's device in order to affect it. Therefore, some people who work with equipment that emits high levels of EMI, such as arc welders, electric drills or hand-held metal detectors, may be able to continue working (35). It would be recommended that the hospital technical staff do field tests measuring the levels of EMI before the patient resumes their job (6).

Other people affected are airline pilots and commercial drivers. The current NASPE and AHA guidelines prohibit aircraft piloting and commercial driving after an ICD has been implanted, but not a pacemaker (35). In Britain, group 2 licence holders will have their commercial licence revoked permanently, even if the ICD is a prophylactic measure (9). Taxi drivers require an individual assessment by the DVLA before they can resume driving commercially. This loss of work can have not only a financial impact but also a loss of self-esteem. Patients will need advice as well as practical support, such as explaining the benefit system to them (5).

IMPLANTABLE CARDIOVERTER DEFIBRILLATOR-RELATED FEARS

Most patients with ICDs fear receiving shocks (26). The most frequently asked questions by patients and their families are what to expect in terms of sensation when the ICD does eventually discharge and whether anybody in contact with the patient at the instant of discharge will feel anything (19). It is important to reassure them that people who touch the patient as the ICD discharges do not get hurt; at most, they feel a slight buzz or tingling (20).

The sensations that people feel when the device discharges vary. Some patients experience warning symptoms, such as dizziness or palpitations, before the device fires, but others receive no warning (26). Patient perceptions of the discharge vary from none to very painful. Patients have described the pain as being like a strong blow to the chest, 'occurring rapidly and without any after effects' to 'a lightning-like blow to the chest' or like being 'kicked in the chest by a horse' (26). Patients with VF or a rapid VT are usually unconscious by the time the ICD discharges. Patients revive immediately, reporting feelings of well-being (20).

Furthermore, many patients who have received shocks exhibit symptoms of classical conditioning by associating specific physical activities or environment with the ICD discharge. They then start avoiding those activities or places, in case the ICD goes off again. This can adversely affect the quality of their life by self-imposed restrictions. In addition, this often leads to diminished self-esteem, heightened concern about their health and decreased independence (26). Patients should be encouraged to revisit a place where the ICD discharged or resume the activity, to avoid this.

ANGER

Anger is seen in many ICD patients, especially those with type A personalities. Levels of anger are higher in patients who have received shocks than in those who have not (26). Heller *et al.* (1998) found that patients who are angry are more likely to view their ICD discharges as 'predominantly negative event[s]' (13).

SYMPTOMS OF DEPRESSION OR SADNESS

Symptoms of depression or sadness, severe enough to affect the quality of life, are reported in up to 58% of patients. Increased sadness was associated with more frequent ICD shocks. Patients may experience 'learned helplessness' – a feeling of hopelessness that can result from having no control over the painful ICD shocks. In many patients, this leads to pessimism about their health status and to depression; these often manifest as reduced sexual activity and fatigue (26). Follow-up support and talking to other ICD recipients have proven to be helpful. However, referral to a psychiatric specialist or antidepressant drugs may be necessary if other measures fail (26).

PHANTOM SHOCK

One manifestation of an emotional response to the ICD has been termed the 'phantom shock' phenomenon (10). This is when patients may think that they have received a shock, but when the ICD is interrogated, there is no record that a discharge has occurred. Phantom shocks are fairly common, often occurring as the patient is drifting off to sleep. It is important to spend time reassuring the patient and family and reviewing the interrogated follow-up printouts with them (20). Phantom shocks seem to be reported more frequently in the first 6 months after implant (10).

An important factor for ICD acceptance is time. Using qualitative data, Burke (1996) described three stages of adjustment: choosing to live life with technology, integrating technology, and living life through technology (8). Quality of life improved when the patient had moved to the last phase of acceptance (10). Despite recurring fear and anxiety, patients usually report a higher quality of life 6 months after receiving an ICD because they have a sense of hope and security for the future (10).

WHAT HAPPENS WHEN THE DEVICE GOES OFF?

On discharge, patients are advised that a single shock is not an emergency – that it just means that the device is working appropriately and they should contact their local outpatient clinic during working hours. They can do this by phone, as many devices can be interrogated by telemetry, and the technician may ask them to put the phone over the device in order to evaluate it. If the shock was appropriate, they can be reassured on the phone without the need for them to attend the hospital.

However, multiple or successive shocks may indicate that the device may be firing inappropriately and should be considered a medical emergency. The patient should be advised to come straight to hospital to have the device evaluated (20).

The ICD is interrogated first to see whether it is delivering appropriate therapy. Approximately 20% of patients with ICDs that use the heart rate only as a detection criterion receive an inappropriate shock. This is usually triggered by atrial fibrillation or sinus tachycardia. However, newer devices with a detection enhancement criterion have helped to reduce this problem considerably. Other causes of inappropriate shocks, especially if the patient is not having clinical symptoms, include dislodged lead, fractured lead or double counting of QRS and T waves (20). Interrogating the ICD's ECG will reveal whether an atrial arrhythmia or lead artifact caused the inappropriate shocks. A chest x-ray can help to diagnose a lead fracture or displacement (20).

In an emergency situation, the ICD can be deactivated by placing a large ICD/pacemaker magnet over the ICD. The magnet suspends the tachycardia detection and inhibits therapy on all ICD devices. Some devices may be permanently placed in the inactive mode with a magnet, and therefore all ICDs should be interrogated whenever a magnet has been placed over the device. Magnets do not inhibit the bradycardia therapy that is programmed into the ICD (20). Patients should be advised to avoid wearing clothing and accessories containing magnets (3).

INVESTIGATIONS PRIOR TO INSERTION OF AN
IMPLANTABLE CARDIOVERTER DEFIBRILLATOR

In order to assess whether somebody is suitable for an ICD, they will have to undergo some investigations. The preliminary, non-invasive investigations, such as physical examination, ECG, chest x-ray, echocardiogram and coronary angiogram, to exclude any underlying coronary disease factors which may require specific treatment and, if specifically requested, a VT stimulation study, can be carried out on an out-patient basis (19).

A VT stimulation is a form of electrophysiological study in which an attempt is made to induce the tachyarrhythmia by programmed electrical stimulation (19). Concerns have been raised about their prognostic value, so they are rarely performed.

POSITION OF AN IMPLANTABLE CARDIOVERTER
DEFIBRILLATOR

Most ICDs can now be implanted in a similar fashion to permanent pacemakers. However, use of the left pectoral region is preferred, so that the heart is central to the vector of the defibrillation current (20). Although successful defibrillation can be achieved with a right-sided implant, it may have an effect on the defibrillation threshold (6).

As the electrical energy is being administered directly to the heart, ICDs require much lower electrical energy to succeed than external defibrillation. Shocks of 10–20 joules are generally sufficient to defibrillate the heart and restore sinus rhythm (17). This is known as the defibrillation threshold (DFT), and is defined as the lowest energy level required to achieve defibrillation (2). One method of lowering DFT is by improving defibrillation waveforms, which describe the manner with which the energy is delivered across the myocardium (2). These waveforms travel from a negatively charged cathode to a positively charged anode. Defibrillation leads may have two shocking coils (one an anode, the other a cathode) (2). Alternately, the ICD generator itself can serve as the fibrillation anode, giving rise to the term *active can* or *hot can*. As the ICD generator has a large surface area, it can provide a more even electrical current distribution and, thus, the DFT can be lower (2).

IMPLANTING AN IMPLANTABLE CARDIOVERTER
DEFIBRILLATOR

The original ICDs were large, which meant that they needed to be implanted in a subcutaneous abdominal pocket. The leads were tunnelled subcutaneously to epicardial patches which were sewn onto the myocardium, thus requiring surgery for their placement. However, by the early 1990s, the size of the pulse generator had decreased sufficiently to allow pectoral implantation (2). Modern ICD pulse generators are now less than half the original size and measure approximately 0.5 inches thick and 2 inches wide (10).

Nowadays, the procedure for ICD insertion is similar to that of a permanent pacemaker and it may be inserted in a cardiac catheterisation laboratory (cath lab). Occasionally, a patient who requires other surgery, such as coronary artery bypass, may have the device implanted in the operating room (4).

Normally, the ICD is implanted subcutaneously in the deltopectoral area under local anaesthesia, with the leads introduced to the heart via the cephalic or sub-clavian veins (29). The device can be implanted subpectorally in thin patients to prevent the device's eroding the skin. However, this location may be asso-ciated with increased complications of bleeding, damage of the thoracoacromial nerves and pectoralis major atrophy, as well as discomfort due to muscle sliding over the pulse generator (2). As with permanent pacemaker placement, abdominal implants are now usually only used in patients in whom a pectoral implant would carry significant risks of pocket erosion, in patients with previous multiple pec-toral pocket infections or in patients whose anatomy precludes pectoral implants. The leads are still introduced into the heart using a transvenous approach (2).

However, unlike the implanting of a permanent pacemaker, the ICD implanta-tion requires induction of ventricle fibrillation to ensure that the arrhythmia can be both detected and terminated by the device. This is carried out under sedation or general anaesthesia to minimise patient discomfort from the shock (17).

HOW THE IMPLANTABLE CARDIOVERTER DEFIBRILLATOR IS TESTED

Through a programmer, the ICD can be used to non-invasively stimulate an arrhythmia, to determine the device's ability to terminate that arrhythmia with its programmed anti-tachycardia therapy. In principle, it is similar to an electrophys-iological test in stimulating arrhythmias but without the invasive introduction of catheters. This is referred to as programmed electrical stimulation (PES) (20). It can also be used to ascertain the integrity of the shocking coil if a lead problem is suspected and for defining the DFT of a patient. For the sake of patient safety, the ICD should be capable of delivering at least 10 joules above the patient's DFT (20).

WHAT A PATIENT CAN EXPECT WHEN UNDERGOING AN IMPLANTABLE CARDIOVERTER DEFIBRILLATOR INSERTION

PRIOR TO THE PROCEDURE

As implanting an ICD is very similar to implanting a pacemaker, the patient should be prepared for the procedure in a similar manner (see Chapter 11).

However, as general anaesthetic or heavy sedation may be used when testing the ICD box, the patients should be advised to fast for 4–6 hours before the procedure (2; 28). Therefore, prior to the procedure, the patient will be assessed by an anaesthetist, who will take a detailed history, looking at issues such as past medical history, chronic illness, reaction to previous anaesthetics and current state of health (27). A combination of inhalational and intravenous anaesthetics may be used. Intravenous agents produce a rapid induction for the patient, which is more pleasant than breathing through a mask, whilst inhalational agents provide maintenance of anaesthesia. Although the inhalational agents are excreted through the lungs, allowing rapid emergence from unconsciousness, the intravenous agents need to be metabolised and excreted by the body, so patients may be drowsy when returning to the ward (27). The anaesthetist may prescribe a pre-medication to reduce anxiety and produce some sedation (18). These should be administered 45–70 minutes prior to the procedure, but only after the consent form has been signed, as they can make a patient drowsy (18).

To minimise bleeding, patients may be asked to stop their antiplatelet medication, such as aspirin, for up to 1 week before the procedure (2). If they are on warfarin, this should be discontinued for at least 4 days before implantation, as their international normalised ratio (INR) should be less than 1.5 (2). If they are at high risk of a thromboembolic event, they may have to be admitted for intravenous heparin therapy while the effects of the warfarin wane (6).

DURING THE PROCEDURE

Once the patient has been positioned on the table, cardiac-monitoring leads will be attached to their torso. As meticulous sterile technique should be exercised throughout the procedure, once the patient is lying on the catheterisation table, they will feel the nursing staff clean the implant area with an iodine/antiseptic solution. Then, the area will be draped with sterile towels (2). Once the patient is prepared, a local anaesthetic (1% lignocaine) will be liberally introduced into the area to be incised. If required, intravenous benzodiazepine (e.g. midazolam) and a narcotic (e.g. fentanyl) can be administered to reduce both anxiety and discomfort. The drugs should be short-acting to minimise the risk of severe respiratory depression (2).

A variety of veins are available for gaining venous access. The cephalic vein cut-down approach is preferred, as venous access is achieved under direct visualisation and there is no risk of pneumothorax. In addition, some believe that there is a lower incidence of lead fraction due to crushing at the junction between the first rib and the clavicle (2). Alternatively, the axillary vein or subclavian vein can be used (2). The subclavian approach is now widely used and is especially useful if more than one lead is to be inserted. As the puncture of the subclavian vein is easier if the vein is distended, patients should be informed that the table may be tilted so that they will be in a slightly head-down position or, alternatively, that their legs may be raised (3). Since the subclavian puncture is performed without direct visualisation of the vein, there is a risk of pneumothorax and subclavian artery puncture (2).

Pacemaker leads are intentionally designed to be flexible to help prevent cardiac perforation. Therefore, once venous access has been achieved, a guidewire is used to help insert the leads into position. When the leads are being positioned, the patient may be asked to stop breathing briefly (without taking a deep breath first), in order to minimise the risk of an air embolism (2).

The ventricular lead is implanted first. Ventricular ectopy is common during lead manipulation and almost always stops when the lead position is stable. Patients should be warned that they may feel a funny sensation in their chest at this time. If VT persists, the lead should be repositioned. If VT continues still, appropriate steps will be taken to terminate the rhythm (2). The atrial lead is implanted next (2).

After satisfactory positions for both leads are found, the leads will be examined under fluoroscopy. During this examination, the patient will be asked to breathe deeply and cough vigorously to ensure that the lead tips are not dislodged by these actions. Pacing at high output should be performed to ensure that there is no pacing of the diaphragm, particularly by the atrial lead, since the right phrenic nerve courses along the lateral right atrium. Once good positioning of both leads has been confirmed, the leads are anchored using a strong non-absorbable suture (2).

An important part of the ICD implantation procedure that is not part of pacemaker implantation is the testing of the device to determine DFT. This is generally performed before closing the wound, after satisfactory lead positions and parameters are obtained. As VF is normally induced deliberately, and a low-energy shock is administered to ensure that all connections are intact, the patient may be sedated or given a general anaesthetic while the device is being tested. The testing is usually performed through a programmer, with a sterile programming wand placed over the implanted pulse generator. Occasionally, testing may be performed through an emulator, which substitutes for the actual pulse generator and connects the defibrillation lead to the programmer. This allows for the decision regarding the ICD model used to be made after the DFT is determined (2).

Once the tests are completed, a subcutaneous or submuscular pocket is made with blunt and sharp dissection and then, depending on the consultant's preference, irrigated liberally with antibiotic solution. The system is then implanted into the pocket, with the lead(s) coiled behind the generator to minimise the risk of damage to the leads in the event of re-incision. The ECG monitor is then examined to ensure appropriate pacing and sensing. The pocket is then closed using two layers of an absorbable suture adhesive tape (such as steri-strips) placed over the incision and then a gauze dressing is placed over the area (2). In order to minimise haematoma formation in the incision site, some patients may have a drain inserted and/or have a pressure dressing applied (25).

POST-PROCEDURE CARE

Similarly to a successful pacemaker implantation, the primary risk in the early post-ICD implantation period is lead displacement. Therefore, patients are advised to remain on bed rest overnight and the arm adjacent to where the ICD is inserted may be put in a sling to restrict movement (2). Whilst the patient is on bed rest, they should be attached to a continuous cardiac monitor to observe for the development of ventricular arrhythmias. If the patient experiences a sustained VT and no therapy is delivered, it is an indication that the programmed detection rate may be above the rate of the tachycardia. A patient with an ICD who has a sustained, haemodynamically unstable rhythm should not be treated any differently from one without an ICD. External cardioversion can be given in an emergency in the absence of therapy from the patient's ICD. Care should be taken not to apply paddles near or above the ICD generator (20).

In addition to cardiac monitoring, 4-hourly temperature, pulse and respiration rates should be recorded (14). If a drain has been inserted, this should be checked regularly and emptied when required. In order to reduce the risk of infection, the drain should be handled as little as possible, and an aseptic technique used when doing so (25).

As the operative approach is almost identical to that of pacemaker implantation, the complications that might be expected with pacemaker implantation can also be encountered after ICD implantation (20) (see Chapter 13); therefore, nurses should observe for:

- signs of infection;
- surgical emphysema around the ICD insertion site; air enters the subcutaneous tissue and it feels crunchy under your fingertips;
- pectoral muscle twitching or hiccups that occur in synchrony with the pacemaker;
- cardiac tamponade; signs and symptoms include persistent hiccups, distant heart sounds, a drop in the strength of a pulse during inspiration, hypotension with a narrowed pulse pressure, cyanosis, distended jugular veins, decreased urine output, restlessness, complaints of a full chest;
- pneumothorax; signs and symptoms include shortness of breath, restlessness and hypoxia; mental status changes and arrhythmias may also occur; diminished breath sounds, usually on the apex of the lung on the side in which the pacemaker was implanted (4); a pneumothorax can normally be seen on a chest x-ray (20).

Anticoagulation should be withheld for several hours to minimise the risk of bleeding and haematoma in the pacemaker pocket (2). In suitable patients, warfarin should be restarted on the evening of the implantation rather than continuing with heparin (29).

As the ICD implant site may be bruised, swollen and tender, especially if a sub-muscular pocket was created, prescribed analgesia should be administered (32) with the prophylactic antibiotics (2).

The drain is usually removed the day after the procedure. As with all drains, it should be removed when the drainage has stopped. First, ensure that any vacuum or suction in the drain is released. Then, using an aseptic technique, the retaining suture should be cut and removed. Using gentle pressure, the drain should be withdrawn. If it does not come out easily, inform the medical staff, as it may have become entangled with the ICD or the wires. Once removed, a small absorbent dressing should be applied to the drain site and observed for excessive amounts of leakage until healing has occurred (25).

The incision site should be inspected for signs of bleeding or infection and the patient informed about how to care for it. Although wounds closed with steri-strips do not normally need an absorbent dressing to cover them, considering where the site is, some patients prefer one to prevent their clothing from irritating the wound (especially ladies wearing bras or men wearing braces).

When the subclavian vein is used, a portable chest x-ray should be taken on the ward on the same day of the procedure to exclude a pneumothorax as well as to verify lead position. No matter which vein is used as access, it is recommended that a posterior–anterior and lateral chest x-ray is to be taken the day after the procedure to examine the stability of lead placement (2).

Before discharge, the pacemaker is interrogated to ensure that no marked changes in lead impedance, pacing threshold or sensing have occurred. Such changes raise the possibility of lead displacement (2). Once it has been established that the leads have not been displaced, the patient is allowed to mobilise.

As patients are normally discharged the day after the procedure, the time available to educate patients and their family is limited; therefore, written discharge instructions should be supplied. This should provide advice about pain management, site assessment and care, what to do in the event of receiving a shock, when to notify the physician, the importance of carrying proper identification that allows medical personnel quickly to check the ICD with the proper programmer, avoiding magnetic fields and, if possible, information regarding support groups (20).

DISCHARGE ADVICE

Upon discharge, patients should be advised:

1. Keep the incision site dry; wait until the third day before having a shower (32).
2. Avoid raising the arm adjacent to the incision site for the first week; shirts or cardigans that button at the front are easier to put on (32).
3. For 1–2 months, do not lift, push or pull anything that weighs more than 5 pounds (2.3 kg), including groceries and children (32).
4. For 1–2 months, avoid arm exercises or activities, like sweeping, that require repeated movement of the arm (32).
5. Do not put pressure on the incision site, such as by wearing braces or tight clothes, until the incision has healed (32).

6. Avoid wearing clothing and accessories containing magnets (3).
7. People with ICDs are still legally required to wear seatbelts but, until the incision has healed, they may find it more comfortable to wear it across the shoulder opposite the incision site.
8. Do not drive until advised to by the cardiologist (32).
9. Tell your other healthcare professionals, such as your dentist, that you have had an ICD inserted (32).
10. Always carry the ICD identification card (32).
11. Vigorous contact sports such as rugby, boxing or judo should be avoided in order to avoid injury to the device (29).
12. An ICD may set off metal detectors or some anti-theft devices, so people with ICDs should carry their ICD identification card to show authorities, if required (32).
13. Inform your cardiologist if there:
    • is any recurrence of your previous symptoms (32);
    • is any sign of infection in the incision site, such as swelling, fluid, pain, redness (or other unusual colour at the pacemaker site), chills or a temperature of 38 °C or higher (32);
    • are hiccups that last more than 15 minutes (32).

When providing the discharge advice, the opportunity should be used to disabuse patients and their families/carers about common misconceptions about ICDs arising from popular notions or outdated information (see Chapter 13).

COMPLICATIONS

As the ICD is placed transvenously, with the pulse generator in the pectoral position, the implantation technique and related complications are the same as those for pacemaker implantation, with the exception that complications can arise as a result of determining the DFT (6). Most patients undergoing ICD implantation will have some discomfort at the site of the incision in the early postoperative period. Mild analgesics may be required (6). The rarer complications can be divided into those that may occur whilst implanting the ICD and those that may occur after the system is in place (20) (see Table 12.1). Nursing staff should be aware of all the potential complications, especially the early ones, so that they know what to look for post procedure. These are discussed in more detail in Chapter 13.

FOLLOW-UP CARE

Patients will be followed up every 3–6 months at outpatient clinic, to assess their clinical status and to review stored data that provide diagnostic information for treated episodes of tachyarrhythmia. The battery status is monitored at each follow-up visit (20). Modern ICDs contain lithium batteries that can last up to 6 years, depending on how often the patient is shocked or whether any of the

Table 12.1. Potential complications of implantable cardioverter defibrillators

Adverse events associated with surgery	Adverse events after system in place
Acceleration of arrhythmia	Chronic nerve damage
Air embolism	Diaphragmatic stimulation
Bleeding	Erosion of pulse generator
Hemothorax	Pocket hematoma
Perforation of the myocardium	Fluid accumulation/seroma
Pneumothorax	Infection of the pocket or system
Puncture of subclavian artery	Keloid formation
Thromboemboli	Lead dislodgment
Venous occlusion	Lead fractures and insulation breaks
	Venous thrombosis

Source: Woods *et al.* (2000) *Cardiac Nursing 4E*. Reproduced by permission of Lippincott, Williams and Wilkins, London.

tiered therapy features are used. One unique feature that an ICD pulse generator has that a pacemaker does not is a beeper that is activated when the battery is low or the ICD has a problem. This audible beep can be heard by both the patient and other people (10).

CARE PLANS

PROBLEM/NEED

Patient is to have an ICD inserted.

PRE-PROCEDURE CARE PLAN FOR PATIENTS UNDERGOING AN ICD IMPLANTATION

Goal/aim of care

Patient to be prepared for ICD insertion, ensuring pre, peri and post-procedure safety.

Action	Rationale
Obtain a brief history and check that biographical details and next of kin are correct	Checking the patient's biographical details and next of kin ensures that medical records are up-to-date and, in the event of an emergency, the correct person is contacted. Record keeping is a fundamental part of nursing care, ensuring high standards of clinical care, and improving communication and dissemination of information (23)

Action	Rationale
Explain the procedure to the patient and significant others, to alleviate anxieties	The period before any procedure may cause extreme anxiety in some patients. Discussion and reassurance may help to relieve some of these feelings (15)
Check whether the patient is allergic to any food, drugs or other substances. Inform the doctor if the patient is allergic to any potential drugs used in the procedure	Patients with a history of allergy to iodine-containing substances, such as seafood or contrast agents, should be given an antihistamine and steroids before the procedure (34). In addition to this, a non-ionic contrast dye may be used for the procedure (6)
Warfarin should be stopped at least 48 hours prior to the procedure	Warfarin should be withheld for at least 48 hours prior to the procedure to ensure an INR of less than 1.5. Patients at high risk of thromboembolism should be admitted for heparinisation while the effects of oral anticoagulation wane (6)
If the patient is normally on warfarin, an INR should be checked prior to the procedure. Aim for an INR of 1.0–1.5	Warfarin interferes with blood coagulation by blocking the effect of vitamin K. It has a long-acting half-life of 36–42 hours. The anticoagulation effect is described in a measurement of the INR. Therefore, any INR measurement of more than 1.5 increases the patient's risk of bleeding uncontrollably during and/or after the procedure (7)
Check that the patient has stopped their antiplatelet medication for at least 1 week prior to the procedure, when appropriate	To minimise bleeding during the procedure (2)
Ensure that the patient has fasted for at least 4–6 hours prior to the procedure	Fasting reduces the risk of aspiration when under general anaesthetic, and eliminates nausea and vomiting post procedure (28; 33)
Obtain baseline blood pressure, pulse, temperature, respiration rate and blood glucose	In order to provide a baseline, for comparison after the ICD has been inserted (14)

Action	Rationale
Record the patient's height and weight	The amount of some of the drugs prescribed during the procedure may be calculated on the patient's body weight (2; 18)
Cannulate the patient	To provide intravenous access to administer prescribed drugs (2; 34)
Remove dentures, artificial eyes, contact lenses and prosthetics	These items may cause confusion when the anaesthetist is assessing the unconscious patient (22)
Ensure that identification and allergy bands are correct, legible and secure	To ensure correct identification and prevent possible problems (34)
If it is not against the patient's religious beliefs, ensure that the skin is shaved where they intend to insert the ICD	Body hair is removed in order to reduce infection risk (34)
Encourage the patient to empty their bladder prior to taking the pre-medication/procedure	To help make them more comfortable (34)
Ensure that the informed consent has been signed prior to the procedure	The procedure and its risks should be explained, and the patient's questions should be answered before the procedure (2)
If the patient is a female of child-bearing age, she may be asked by the radiographer to sign a form indicating her pregnancy status	Pregnancy is a relative contraindicator in cardiac intervention procedures (16). However, as direct irradiation of the uterus can usually be avoided in procedures that involve structures above the diaphragm, fluoroscopic procedures on pregnant women may be justifiable in an emergency situation (2)

POST-PROCEDURE CARE PLAN

Goal/aim of care

The nursing care of patients following ICD insertion is directed towards the prevention and detection of complications.

Action	Rationale
Attach the patient to a cardiac monitor and check blood pressure and pulse	The heart rhythm should be monitored after ICD insertion to observe for ventricular arrhythmias and whether the ICD is responding appropriately to them. In addition, if the ICD has a combined function and is acting as pacemaker, or providing CRT, the heart rhythm should be monitored to ensure that it is pacing properly (2; 14)
Check blood pressure and temperature every 4 hours post procedure	In order to observe for any haemodynamic compromise (14)
Pulse oximetry	Hypoxia occurs for a variety of reasons following anaesthesia. The administration of supplemental oxygen in the immediate post-operative phase will help to reduce the risk of hypoxia's occurring. The aim is to maintain normal levels of arterial blood gases and peripheral oxygen saturations (27)
Respiratory rate	Anaesthesia and opiates may depress respiration. Although the anaesthetist aims to have reversed these effects by the time the patient is warded, there is potential for severe respiratory depression to be present in the immediate post-procedure period (27)
If the patient is a diabetic, check their blood sugar on warding	To ensure that the patient is not hypoglycaemic, as they may have fasted for long periods prior to the procedure (34)
Ensure that the sedation/anaesthetic has worn off prior to providing something to drink or eat. Try the patient with sips of water initially	If the patient is not fully conscious before eating or drinking, they may inhale it (33)
Ensure that any intravenous fluids are running at the correct rate, and administer any drugs prescribed post procedure	It is the ward nurses' responsibility to ensure that the prescribed drugs, intravenous or oral, are administered correctly (20; 24)

Action	Rationale
If a drain was inserted, regularly check and empty the drain	To minimise haematoma formation (25)
If the subclavian vein was utilised, obtain a portable chest x-ray on the ward	It is difficult to identify a pneumothorax or haemothorax on a chest x-ray when the patient is lying down; therefore, the patient should have an upright chest x-ray when the subclavian vein is used (2)
Advise patients to take things slowly when they first mobilise	A patient may drop their blood pressure by simply standing up abruptly after prolonged bed rest (31)
Prior to discharge, re-dress the incision and look for signs of weeping, redness or inflammation	To check for signs of excessive bleeding or infection (2; 14)
Discharge home with both verbal and written advice	Discharge information should be given in both written and verbal forms, ensuring that patients understand this prior to leaving (14)
Any changes in medication should be discussed with the patient	When discharging a patient, it is the nurses' responsibility to inform the patient about the medication that they have been prescribed so that they will take it correctly at home (24)

Driving restrictions

Driving restrictions associated with ICDs vary and depend on why the ICD was implanted, if and when they had a shockable rhythm and their level of heart failure.

No matter the reason for the ICD implantation, all group 2 drivers are permanently barred from driving. Group 2 includes large lorries and buses. The medical standards for group 2 drivers are much higher than those for group 1 because of the size and weight of the vehicle and also the length of time that the driver may spend at the wheel in the course of their occupation (9).

Non-commercial group 1 drivers are split into the following three categories.

Prophylactic implantable cardioverter defibrillator implant

- Symptomatic individuals who have a high risk of significant arrhythmia are prohibited from driving for 1 month after ICD implantation.

- They do not need to inform the DVLA.
- However, if the ICD subsequently delivers ATP and/or shock therapy (except during normal clinical testing), they are not allowed to drive for 6 months and the DVLA should be notified (9).

Implantable cardioverter defibrillator implanted for ventricular arrhythmia which did not cause incapacity

If the patient presents with a non-disqualifying cardiac event, namely haemodynamically stable non-incapacitating VT, the patient does not need to inform the DVLA and can drive 1 month after implantation if all the following conditions are met:

1. LVEF greater than 35%.
2. No fast VT induced on electrophysiological study (RR < 250 milliseconds).
3. Any induced VT could be pace-terminated by the ICD twice without acceleration during the post-implantation study.

If all these criteria cannot be met, then these patients cannot drive for 6 months and the DVLA need to be informed. In addition, should the ICD subsequently deliver ATP and/or shock therapy (except during normal clinical testing), they are not allowed to drive for 6 months and the DVLA should be notified (9).

Implantable cardioverter defibrillator implanted for ventricular arrhythmia which did cause incapacity

Patients should inform the DVLA following the initial ICD implantation and should not drive for:

1. A period of 6 months after the first implant.
2. A further 6 months after any shock therapy and/or symptomatic anti-tachycardia pacing (see 3a below).
3. A period of 2 years if any therapy following device implantation has been accompanied by incapacity (whether caused by the device or arrhythmia) except for:

   3a. If therapy was delivered due to an inappropriate cause, i.e. atrial fibrillation or programming issues, then driving may resume 1 month after this has been completely controlled to the satisfaction of the cardiologist, in which case the DVLA will need to be notified.

   3b. If the incapacitating shock was appropriate (i.e. for sustained VT or VF) and new therapy has to be introduced to prevent recurrence, driving may resume after 6 months in the absence of further symptomatic therapy.
4. A period of 1 month off driving must occur following any revision of the electrodes or alteration of antiarrhythmic drug treatment.
5. A period of 1 week off driving is required after a defibrillator box change (9).

For patients who fall into categories 2 and 3, if the patient has been re-licensed prior to the event, the DVLA should be informed.

Resumption of driving requires that:

1. The device is subject to regular review with interrogation.
2. There is no other disqualifying condition (9).

REFERENCES

1. Al-Obaidi, M., Noble, M. and Siva, A. (2004) *Crash Course Cardiology*, 2nd edn, London, Mosby.
2. Baim, D. S. and Grossman, W. (2000) *Grossman's Cardiac Catheterisation: Angiography, and Intervention*, 6th edn, London, Lippincott Williams & Wilkins.
3. Bennett, D. H. (2002) *Cardiac Arrhythmias: Practical Notes on Interpretation and Treatment*, London, Arnold.
4. Beverage, D., Haworth, K., Labus, D., Mayer, B. and Munson, S. (2005) *ECG Interpretation Made Incredibly Easy*, London, Lippincott Williams & Wilkins.
5. Bowles, C. (2002) 'Shock to the system', *Nursing Standard*, 16(38): 16–19.
6. Braunwald, E., Zipes, D. and Libby, P. (2001) *Heart Disease: A Textbook of Cardiovascular Medicine*, 6th edn, Philadelphia, PA, W.B. Saunders Co.
7. Blann, A., Landray, M. and Lip, G. (2002) 'An overview of antithrombotic therapy', *British Medical Journal*, 325: 762–5.
8. Burke, I. J. (1996) 'Securing life through technology acceptance: The first six months after internal cardioverter defibrillator implantation', *Heart Lung*, 25: 352–66.
9. DVLA (2006) *For Medical Practitioners: At a Glance Guide to the Current Medical Standards for Fitness to Drive*, February, available online at *www.dvla.gov.uk*.
10. Fetzer, S. J. (2003) 'The patient with an implantable cardioverter defibrillator', *Journal Peri-Anaesthesia Nursing*, 18(6): 398–405.
11. Frodsham, R. (2005) 'Cardiac resynchronisation therapy for patients with heart failure', *Nursing Standard*, 19(45): 46–50.
12. Hamilton, G. and Carroll, G. (2004) 'The effects of age on quality of life in implantable cardioverter defibrillator recipients', *Journal of Clinical Nursing*, 13: 194–200.
13. Heller, S. S., Ormont, M. A., Lidagoster, L., Sciacca, R. R. and Steinberg, J. S. (1998) 'Psychosocial outcome after ICD implantation: A current perspective', *Pacing Clinical Electrophysiological*, 21(6): 1207–15.
14. Hubbard, J. (2003) 'An overview of permanent and temporary cardiac pacemakers', *Nursing Times*, 99(36): 26–7.
15. Hughes, S. (2002) 'The effects of pre-operative information', *Nursing Standard*, 16(28): 33–7.
16. Kern, M. (2003) *The Cardiac Catheterisation Handbook*, 4th edn, London, Mosby.
17. Julian, D., Cowan, J. C. and McLenachan, J. M. (2005) *Cardiology*, 8th edn, Edinburgh, Elsevier Saunders.
18. Lemone, P. and Burke, K. (2004) *Medical/Surgical Nursing: Critical Thinking in Client Care*, 3rd edn, Upper Saddle River, NJ, Prentice Hall.
19. Moon, M. (2001) Implantation of implantable defibrillators: Implication for nursing practice', *Nursing in Critical Care*, 6(3): 133–8.
20. Morton, P., Fontaine, D., Hudak, C. and Gallo, B. (2005) *Critical Care Nursing: A Holistic Approach*, 8th edn, Philadelphia, PA, Lippincott Williams & Wilkins.

21. NICE (2006) 'Implantable cardioverter defibrillators for arrhythmias: Review of Technology Appraisal 11', available online at *www.nice.org.uk/ta.095*.
22. Norell, M. and Perrins, J. (2003) *Essential Interventional Cardiology*, Philadelphia, PA, W.B. Saunders Co.
23. Nursing Midwifery Council (2002a) *Guidelines for Records and Record Keeping*, London, Nursing and Midwifery Council, April.
24. Nursing Midwifery Council (2002b) *Guidelines for the Administration of Medicines*, London, Nursing and Midwifery Council.
25. Pudner, R. (2000) *Nursing the Surgical Patient*, London, Bailliere Tindall.
26. Shaffer, R. S. (2002) 'ICD therapy: The patient's perspective', *American Journal Nursing*, **102**(2): 46–9.
27. Sheppard, M. and Wright, M. (2000) *Principles and Practice of High Dependency Nursing*, Edinburgh, Bailliere Tindall.
28. Soreide, E., Eriksson, L. I., Hirlekar, G., Eriksson, H., Henneberg, W., Sandin, R. and Raeder, J. (Task Force on Scandinavian Pre-operative Fasting Guidelines, Clinical Practice Committee Scandinavian Society of Anaesthesiology and Intensive Care Medicine) (2005) 'Pre-operative fasting guidelines: An update', *Acta Anaesthesiologica Scandinavica*, **49**: 1041–7.
29. Swanton, R. H. (2003) *Cardiology*, 5th edn, Malden, MA, Blackwell Publishing.
30. Tagney, J. (2004) 'Can nurses in cardiology areas prepare patients for implantable cardioverter defibrillator implant and life at home?', *Nursing in Critical Care*, **9**(3): 104–14.
31. Topol, E. J. (1999) *Textbook of Interventional Cardiology*, 3rd edn, London, W.B. Saunders Co.
32. Toth, P. and Knect, J. (2004) 'Pacemakers', *Nursing*, **34**(1): 46–7.
33. Webb, K. (2003) 'What are the benefits and the pitfalls of preoperative fasting?', *Nursing Times*, **99**(50): 32–3, available online at *wwwnursingtimes.net*.
34. Woods, S., Froelicher, E. and Motzer, S. (2000) *Cardiac Nursing*, 4th edn, Philadelphia, PA, Lippincott Williams & Wilkins.
35. Yeo, T. P. (2004) 'Counselling patients with implanted cardiac devices', *The Nurse Practitioner*, **29**(12): 58–65.

13 Common Problems Associated with Permanent Pacemakers and Implantable Cardioverter Defibrillators

POTENTIAL COMPLICATIONS OF PERMANENT PACEMAKER/IMPLANTABLE CARDIOVERTER DEFIBRILLATOR IMPLANTATION

As the majority of permanent pacemakers (PPMs) and implantable cardioverter defibrillators (ICDs) are implanted in the left pectoral region and the leads introduced transvenously to the heart, complications associated with either procedure are very similar (4). Although the risks associated with transvenous implantation of PPM/ICD are low, complications do occur. Nursing staff should be aware of all the potential complications, especially the early ones, so that they know what to look for post procedure (1).

PAIN

Most patients undergoing PPM/ICD implantation will have some discomfort at the site of the incision in the early post-operative period. Mild analgesics may be required (4).

MILD BRUISING

Mild bruising is not uncommon but, occasionally, poor haemostasis will result in a haematoma (2).

HAEMATOMA

Haematoma formation at the pulse generator site most commonly occurs when anticoagulation therapy is initiated or restarted prematurely. After administering analgesia, manual compression over the haematoma may reduce the tenseness in the haematoma and thus avoids evacuation. However, evacuation of the haematoma should be considered if there is continued bleeding, potential compromise of the suture line or skin integrity, or analgesics are not controlling the pain from the haematoma (4).

PNEUMOTHORAX

As the subclavian vein is close to the top of the lung, there is an increased risk that using this vein for transvenous access may cause a pneumothorax. The symptoms may occur suddenly, or may insidiously present up to 48 hours after the procedure. The symptoms include pleuritic pain, hypotension, respiratory distress or hypoxia. A chest x-ray can reveal the extent of the trauma. Although a small pneumothorax may resolve without intervention (1), when severe, a chest drain may be required to allow for lung re-expansion (see overleaf) (6).

ABDOMINAL TWITCHING OR HICCUPS

The phrenic nerve or the diaphragm can sometimes be stimulated through the intervening thin myocardial walls by atrial and ventricular leads, respectively (2). This complication is usually very uncomfortable for the patient, but can sometimes be corrected by programming the output of the generator to a lower level; otherwise, the leads will need to be repositioned (6). Diaphragmatic stimulation can sometimes be associated with lead perforation. Therefore, the patient should have a chest x-ray and be closely monitored if they drop their blood pressure, in addition to diaphragmatic stimulation, especially if there is a high capture threshold (6).

LEAD DISLODGEMENT/DISPLACEMENT

Lead dislodgement/displacement may result in oversensing, undersensing or failure to capture, and may necessitate repositioning of the leads (6). This was once a common problem, but, with modern leads, it occurs in fewer than 1% of implantations (2). However, as the left-ventricular wall leads in biventricular pacemakers are not anchored in place, it has a higher risk for lead displacement (3). Lead dislodgement is most likely to occur early after implantation (within a day). Therefore, pacemaker interrogation and a chest x-ray are recommended on the day following the procedure (1).

LEAD FRACTURE

With modern leads, fracture is rare. If it does occur, it is usually at the point at which the lead enters the venous system, at the site of a fixation suture or wherever there is excessive angulation of the lead. Lead fracture will cause intermittent or persistent failure to pace and sense. Lead impedance will be markedly elevated. Lead fracture can often be detected by x-ray but should not be confused with 'pseudofracture': when the pressure of a tight ligature is directly applied to the lead, it may compress the insulation and spread the coils of wire inside without interfering with lead function (2).

PERICARDIAL TAMPONADE

There is a small risk of perforating the thin-walled right ventricle or atrium with the leads. Vigilance is necessary and the index of suspicion for pericardial tamponade should be high during and after the procedure. Tamponade may present as an apparent 'vagal' episode. However, as the heart rate will be supported by the pacemaker, the tachycardia that typically accompanies pericardial tamponade may be absent in the pacemaker patient (1). Perforation can be suspected if the patient demonstrates a change in pre-cordial lead morphology on cardiac monitoring (6). Other symptoms include pallor, hypotension, sweating, loss of voltage on ECG and chest pain (9). Pericardial tamponade can be confirmed by an echocardiogram (6). Although small leaks usually repair themselves without complication, if the patient is symptomatic, the pericardial sac must be decompressed to restore adequate cardiac output (9).

INFECTION

Reports of cardiac device infection rates vary between 2 and 8% (12). If there is evidence of systemic infection (fever, positive blood cultures), removal of the entire system (device and lead(s)) is indicated, to allow antibiotic therapy to clear the infection completely (1). PPM/ICD infection may appear as local inflammation or abscess formation in the PPM/ICD pocket, erosion of part of the pacing system with secondary infection, or sepsis with positive blood culture findings with or without focus of infection elsewhere (4).

EROSION

Erosion is a late complication but is often a consequence of implantation technique. Factors that predispose to erosion include creation of a PPM/ICD pocket which is too tight or too superficial, a very thin patient and use of a device with sharp corners. The skin will be found to be thinned around the site of erosion. Infection is often present but it is secondary to erosion. If the skin is broken, explantation will be necessary. Thinned, reddened skin over the generator is a sign of 'threatened' erosion: the box should be resited (2). When a PPM/ICD erodes, an aggressive infection may occur throughout the lead system into the heart, making lead extraction necessary (6).

THE 'TWIDDLER'S SYNDROME'

If the PPM/ICD pocket is too large, the device may rotate spontaneously, or be repeatedly moved by the patient. This can cause lead dislodgement or fracture of the leads. Thus, the leads would need to be repositioned or replaced (2).

SUBCLAVIAN VEIN

As the subclavian vein cannot be visualised by the operator, it is referred to as a blind puncture. As a result, potential complications include pneumothorax and haemothorax, inadvertent arterial puncture, air embolism, arteriovenous fistula, thoracic duct injury, surgical emphysema and brachial plexus injury. Fortunately, these complications are very rare (4).

EXIT BLOCK

The development of excessive fibrous tissue, which is non-excitable, around the electrode may increase the stimulation threshold to a level higher than the pace-maker's output. The result will be intermittent or persistent failure to pace without evidence of lead displacement. Exit block is most likely to occur in the first 3 weeks to 3 months after implantation, when the stimulation threshold is at its highest. Sometimes, the exit block is transient; otherwise, lead repositioning will be required unless generator output can be increased by reprogramming. Modern leads with low surface area, porous-surfaced electrodes, steroid-eluting tips and positive-fixation devices rarely give rise to this complication (2).

VENOUS THROMBOSIS

The development of a thrombosis in the subclavian vein or lungs is a very rare complication. It can be treated with anticoagulation therapy (2).

CHEST DRAIN

As the subclavian vein is close to the top of the lung, puncturing this vein to insert a pacemaker or ICD box may cause a pneumothorax or haemothorax (2; 6). A pneumothorax is the presence of air between the visceral and parietal pleura, while a haemothorax occurs when blood enters the pleural spaces and compresses the lung. This results in loss of an area of the lung for gas exchange and supply of oxygen to the tissues (8). The symptoms may occur suddenly, or may insidiously present up to 48 hours after the procedure. The symptoms include pleuritic pain, hypotension, respiratory distress or hypoxia (6). A pneumothorax or haemothorax can be seen on upright chest x-ray (1). Although a small collection of air may resolve spontaneously within several days (1), in severe cases, a chest drain should be inserted to allow the lung to re-expand (6).

A chest drain works by removing air, fluid or blood from the pleural space, thus restoring the negative pressure in the pleural space which will re-expand a collapsed or partially collapsed lung and prevent reflux of drainage back into the chest (6).

There are several different types of chest drains but the most common system is a one-bottle system (8) (Figure 13.1). This consists of a chest tube which is

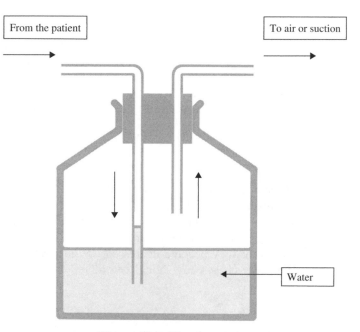

From the patient

To air or suction

Water

Figure 13.1. The chest drain.

inserted into the pleural or mediastinal space of the lung. This is attached to a long tube which is attached to the drainage bottle. The bottle is filled with sterile water to a prescribed level that forms a seal that prevents outside air from entering the system. The drainage bottle can be connected to a suction pump if it is required (6; 8).

To prevent infection, sterile technique should be used when inserting a chest drain, but it can be inserted on the ward by the patient's bedside (6). A chest x-ray must be performed after a chest drain is inserted so that its position can be verified and to assess the degree of re-expansion of the lung and plethora. The x-ray can also enable professionals to assess the amount of residual pleural fluid (8).

POSITIONING THE DRAINAGE BOTTLE AND TUBING

The drainage bottle must be kept below chest level to prevent fluid re-entering the pleural space (8). However, the patient should be encouraged to sit upright and to mobilise. This will increase the use of their lungs, thus enhancing chest expansion. In addition to this, deep breathing and coughing will raise the intra-thoracic pressure and promote pleural drainage. Patients should be educated about moving with a drain to avoid accidental disconnection or kinking of the tubing (8).

Looping the drainage tube should be avoided, as it can impede drainage, thus increasing the pressure in the tubing, which can lead to a tension pneumothorax or surgical emphysema. Therefore, the drainage tubing should be laid horizontally across the bed or chair before dropping it vertically into the drainage bottle (8).

NURSING MANAGEMENT OF A CHEST DRAIN

Nursing care is directed at maintaining patency and proper functioning of the chest-tube drainage system. Vigilant and expert nursing care can prevent serious complications in the patient with a chest tube and drainage system (6). How frequently observations and checks are recorded will vary, depending on the condition of the patient, the amount of fluid expected to be lost and local guidelines (8).

General observations

Observations should include heart rate, blood pressure, temperature and oxygen saturation. If the equipment is available, it is also useful to perform arterial blood gases. Breath sound, chest movement, respiration rate, pattern, depth and effort associated with breathing should also be recorded. If there is any deterioration in the patient's condition or they become distressed, the medical team must be notified at once and another chest x-ray should be ordered (8).

Monitoring the chest drain

At frequent intervals, the chest-drain system should be checked for drainage, suction level and water-seal integrity (6).

Drainage

Maintaining a 24-hour record of drainage will help to determine when a drain may be removed. The colour, consistency and amount of drainage should be recorded regularly (8). A sudden increase in drainage may indicate a haemorrhage or a sudden patency of a previously blocked tube. A sudden decrease indicates that the chest tube is obstructed or failure in the drainage system (6).

The patient should be repositioned to try and alleviate the obstruction. If a clot is visible, straighten the tubing between the chest and the drainage bottle and raise the tube to try and enhance the effect of gravity (6).

Suction level

Low-grade suction can be used to aid the removal of air or fluid from the chest cavity. There is currently no consensus on how much suction should be applied, but the most commonly used pressure is 5 kPa. Too little suction will prevent lung expansion, thus increasing the risk of tension pneumothorax, fluid accumulation and infection. Too much can perpetuate an air leak and cause air stealing, in which the flow through the lung and into the drainage system is too rapid for adequate oxygenation to occur. This can lead to hypoxia and may also result in pieces of lung becoming trapped in the drain (8).

Water-seal integrity

In order to maintain the integrity of the seal in the chest-drain system, it is important that the water level is at least 2 cm above where the chest-tube drain enters the drainage bottle. Because water evaporates over time, especially when suction is being applied, sterile water may have to be added to the drainage bottle to preserve that integrity. The suction will have to be disconnected briefly in order to accurately assess the water level in the chamber (6).

Respiratory fluctuations (referred to as swinging) are observed in the water-seal chamber. The absence of fluctuations can indicate that the lung is re-expanded or that there is an obstruction in the system. Continuous vigorous bubbling in the water-seal chamber, without suction, indicates continued pneumothorax, or it can indicate that the tube has been displaced or disconnected, or that the drainage system is damaged. The entire system should be checked for disconnections and the chest tube inspected to see whether it is displaced outside the chest (6).

Pain management

Having a chest drain can be painful, which may inhibit both the patient's movement and lung expansion and consequently their recovery; therefore, regular analgesia should be administered (8).

Dressings

If a chest drain has been sutured in place correctly, air should not leak from the site and a small, dry non-adherent surgical dressing with an adhesive border should be sufficient. The site should be checked every day and if the dressing is clean and dry, it will need to be changed only every 48–72 hours (8).

Clamping drains

The most serious complication resulting from chest-tube placement is tension pneumothorax, which can develop if there is any obstruction in the chest-tube drainage system. Clamping chest tubes as a routine practice predisposes patients to this complication (6). A tension pneumothorax occurs when the air from the alveoli enters but cannot leave the pleural space. The air can build up, causing a mediastinal shift towards the unaffected lung. This shift compresses the vena cava and is associated with shock and collapse. If bubbling is observed in the underwater seal drain, the chest tube should never be clamped. The drain is allowing the air to escape and, if it is clamped, the air cannot escape and tension pneumothorax will develop (8).

A non-bubbling chest drain should not usually be clamped except momentarily in the event of its being disconnected, if there is damage to the drainage bottle or to locate a leak in the drainage system (8). If the tube must be clamped, padded haemostats should be used to avoid cutting the chest tube (6).

Milking and stripping

Studies have suggested that milking and stripping techniques may not be beneficial for the maintenance of chest-tube patency. These techniques may excessively increase intra-pleural and intra-pulmonary pressure, affecting ventricular function or causing trauma from aspiration of lung tissue into chest-tube eyelets. They also increase the risk of pneumothorax. However, this procedure may be necessary in cases of active bleeding to prevent blood clotting in the tubing that could lead to cardiac or pleural tamponade (6; 8).

Changing the drainage bottle

A one-bottle/one-chamber device is generally adequate to evacuate an uncomplicated pneumothorax, haemothorax or pleural effusion. However, if necessary, the chest tube can be clamped momentarily to change a bottle (8).

REMOVAL OF A CHEST DRAIN

Chest drains are usually removed when drainage is less than 100–150 ml over 24 hours, breath sounds have returned to normal, bubbling in the underwater seal drain has ceased and the chest x-ray shows that the underlying problem has resolved (8).

Removing a chest drain can be a painful procedure, which is often described as a stinging or burning sensation. It is therefore recommended that analgesia should be administered beforehand and be given time to take effect (8).

It normally takes two people to perform this procedure: one to remove the drain, the other to tie the suture to close the wound (8).

One of the main complications associated with removal of a drain is recurrent pneumothorax. This is more likely if the patient breathes in while the drain is being removed, as air can be drawn into the pleural space on inspiration. To prevent this, the patient should be told to take a deep breath and hold it while the drain is being removed (8).

Alternatively, the patient could be asked to perform the Valsalva manoeuvre. This involves increasing the intra-thoracic pressure by holding their breath, while trying to breathe out against a closed glottis. This increases the intra-thoracic pressure, which reduces the possibility of air re-entering the pleural space through the drain site. The drain can be removed while the patient is holding their breath on expiration (8).

A chest x-ray should be performed as soon as the drains are removed to check that a pneumothorax has not recurred, and both the patient and the drain site should be monitored closely (8).

COMPLICATIONS ASSOCIATED WITH A CHEST DRAIN

Tension pneumothorax

The most serious complication resulting from chest-tube placement is tension pneumothorax, which can develop if there is any obstruction in the chest-tube drainage system (6). A tension pneumothorax, which can be life-threatening, occurs when air enters the pleural space during inspiration but cannot escape during expiration. The increasing volume of trapped air collapses the lungs and compresses the soft tissues in the chest. This can occur if the drain is not positioned properly (8).

Surgical emphysema

Surgical emphysema may occur if one or more drainage holes are situated outside the pleural space or if the tubing is blocked or kinked. Surgical emphysema develops because the air cannot escape down the tube and therefore enters the subcutaneous tissue. It causes a crackling noise when the skin is touched, and feels crunchy under your fingertips (3; 8).

Surgical emphysema can make the arms, chest and neck swell and, in severe cases, cause facial swelling to the extent that the patient's eyes may be forced to close. Nothing can be done to reduce the swelling and it may take several days to go down, but inserting an additional chest drain may prevent it from getting worse (8).

Infection

The patient and the chest drain should be assessed at least daily for signs of systemic or local infection. There is a risk that a collection of pus may occur and require prompt treatment. The wound site is also at risk of infection and aseptic procedure should be followed when cleaning the site (8).

Air leak

A large air leak, indicated by continuous bubbling, may suggest that there is a tear at the suture line on the lungs that may need immediate repair. Other causes of air leaks include poor tube connections and a poor seal around the entry site of the drain and these require prompt correction (8).

Other complications

Other complications may include pain, incorrect placement, injury to intercostal muscles, perforation of heart, liver, lung, stomach and aorta (8).

Occasionally, the chest tube may fall out or be accidentally pulled out. In such circumstances, the insertion site should be quickly sealed off using petroleum gauze covered with dry gauze and occlusive tape dressing to prevent air from entering the pleural cavity (6).

EQUIPMENT REQUIRED FOR A CHEST-DRAIN INSERTION

- chest-tube tray or thoracotomy tray (with scalpel);
- chest tube;
- 1% lignocaine;

- antiseptic (povidone-iodine);
- sterile gloves;
- large haemostats;
- suture material (0.0 or 2.0 silk) on a cutting needle;
- bacteriostatic ointment or petroleum gauze;
- sterile gauze with slit;
- tape, both wide and narrow, or an occlusive dressing;
- chest-tube drainage system and suction;
- sterile water for water-seal systems;
- medication for pain and sedation (6).

POTENTIAL MISCONCEPTIONS ABOUT PERMANENT PACEMAKERS/IMPLANTABLE CARDIOVERTER DEFIBRILLATORS

Electromagnetic interference (EMI) is electrical signals from the environment (i.e. radiofrequency waves) that can be sensed by the PPM/ICD and interfere with its function (11). In pacemakers, it may convert an asynchronous mode (demand pacing) to synchronous mode (fixed pacing) (6). In ICDs, it may cause inappropriate shocks, re-programme the ICD parameters, resulting in failure to deliver appropriate anti-tachycardia pacing, and interfere with bradycardic support. Therefore, all PPM/ICDs should be checked and their parameters reset after exposure to EMI (4). Fortunately, experts feel that sources of EMI must be in close proximity (within 6 inches/15 cm) to the patient's device in order to affect it (12). However, patients and their families may have misconceptions about limitations caused by PPM/ICD due to popular notions or outdated information.

Touching the patient

The patient and his/her family should be reassured that as such low doses of electricity are being used, it is safe to touch them when the defibrillator fires. They may feel a slight buzz or tingling, like a static shock, or they may feel the patient's muscle twitch (5; 6).

Cellular phone

There is a possibility that some high-power digital mobile phones may transiently interfere with the PPM/ICD functions. Therefore, people with these devices should be advised to keep a mobile telephone at least 6 inches/15 cm from the device and, when using the phone, to use the ear opposite to the implant site. They should also avoid carrying an activated phone in a pocket that is near the device (4; 10).

Sport

Vigorous contact sports (e.g. rugby, football, soccer, boxing, judo or karate) are best avoided by patients with PPM/ICDs in order to avoid injury to the device. Squash should be discouraged, if possible (7). However, patients can still participate in sports such as golf, tennis or basketball. Pacemaker patients can even participate in more strenuous activities, such as marathons or scuba diving, after consultation with their cardiologists. Any activity restrictions usually result from other medical problems and not from the device (10).

Microwaves and power tools

Some old microwaves caused interference with PPM/ICDs in the past. However, modern microwaves are better shielded nowadays, so people with PPM/ICDs can use all types of household appliances and power tools. However, arc-welding equipment and high-voltage commercial transformers should be avoided (10).

Travelling

By always carrying the identification card given to them at the time of the PPM/ICD implantation, patients can have their device evaluated in almost any part of the world, if required (10). They can also show this card to officials when required. For example, PPM/ICD recipients should avoid security hand-held metal detectors near their device. Hand-held (wand-type) devices contain magnets that can reset the PPM/ICD sensing programs, causing the device to malfunction. It may be safer to ask to walk through a regular security gate or ask to be searched by hand. PPM/ICD recipients can walk briskly through the upright security gates but should avoid pausing in the middle or leaning against the posts (12).

Theft-detector devices

Theft-detector devices will not affect the PPM/ICDs unless there is prolonged exposure (4). However, they may trigger the alarm system as the recipient walks out of the shop. Showing their device's information card will help to explain the situation to shopkeepers (7).

Loud speakers

Very large stereo speakers contain strong magnets that may inhibit pacemakers and interfere with ICDs. Therefore, recipients should keep a reasonable distance from them (7; 12).

Diathermy/electrocautery

Diathermy/electrocautery may damage a pacemaker, causing inappropriate inhibition or possible ventricular fibrillation. The pulse should be monitored throughout the surgery so that diathermy/electrocautery can be interrupted if prolonged inhibition occurs. Ideally, the pacemaker should be checked prior to surgery, as some pacemakers are more prone to external interference when the batteries are approaching end of life. A pacemaker check should be performed soon after surgery (2). ICD recipients should have their device turned off prior to surgery that requires diathermy/electrocautery. The safest method is to turn off its detection mode with a programmer but if one is not available, a ring magnet taped over the ICD box will deactivate it temporarily. The magnet will not affect backup pacing. The ICD parameters should be rechecked once the surgery has been completed (1; 7).

Radiation

For diagnostic purposes, radiation will not affect a PPM/ICD but therapeutic levels may cause damage. The pacemaker should be shielded and, if this is not possible, resiting of the device should be considered (2).

Transcutaneous electrical nerve stimulation (TENS)

As this can affect PPM/ICDs, the patient should be monitored when they have this treatment. If there is evidence of oversensing in the ICD patients, the TENS electrodes must be removed (2; 7).

Magnetic resonance imaging

Magnetic resonance imaging is contraindicated for both PPM and ICD recipients (2; 4).

Lithotripsy

Lithotripsy is contraindicated if the ICD is in the lithotripsy field (4). However, pacemaker patients can avail of this treatment if the shocks are not focused directly over the pacemaker and the pacemaker is programmed to non-rate-responsive VVI mode (2).

Electroconvulsive therapy

It is safe to apply electroconvulsive therapy to patients with a pacemaker (2). However, the ICD should be deactivated for the treatment and the patient monitored for arrhythmias throughout the procedure. The ICD can be reactivated once the treatment session has been completed (5).

Welding

As arc welding emits high levels of EMI, it has generally been considered not suitable for a person with a PPM/ICD. However, some data suggest that some patients can be allowed to carry out this activity if they are evaluated in their work environment (4).

Vibration

Hovercraft, helicopters and other sources of vibration may increase the rate of activity-sensing pacemakers, and therefore lead to inappropriate inhibition (7). If necessary, the patient can switch the pacemaker to a fixed-rate mode by placing a magnet over the device, which renders it immune to external signals. The pacemaker will revert to asynchronous mode once the magnet is removed (7).

Magnet application

Placing a magnet directly over a pacemaker can activate its reed-switch and convert it from pacing in demand mode to a fixed-rate mode. The effect should only last as long as the magnet is applied (2). Once the pacemaker is in fixed-rate mode, it is immune to external signals, and will pace at the prescribed level. Therefore, if the patient is at risk of external interference that may bombard the pacemaker and inhibit its sensing function, and thus fail to pace appropriately, a magnet can be placed over it for the duration. A common example is the use of diathermy/electrocautery for a surgical procedure (1).

A magnet placed over an ICD will suspend tachycardia detection and inhibit shock therapy. It should not inhibit the bradycardia therapy that is programmed into the ICD (6). In an emergency, a ring magnet may be placed over the device to deactivate it. The ICD's response to a magnet is a programmable feature so it might be different depending on the generation, manufacturer and model of the ICD. In some models, an audible beep is heard when a magnet is placed over the device. This is followed by an active tone to indicate that the device is inactive. A patient should be monitored whenever a magnet is used to deactivate the ICD and the ICD checked that its programmed parameters are normal after the magnet has been removed (5).

Patients with a PPM/ICD should be reassured that the magnet needs to be over the device for at least 30 seconds before it will affect it (6). However, they should be advised to avoid clothing and accessories which contain magnets. Other unexpected sources of magnets in accessories include retention clips in jewellery, fasteners for shoulder bags and backpacks, button-hole holders and storage clips for headphones (2; 7).

Cremation

A PPM/ICD must be explanted before cremation, to avoid explosion (2).

REFERENCES

1. Baim, D. S. and Grossman, W. (2000) *Grossman's Cardiac Catheterisation: Angiography and Intervention*, 6th edn, London, Lippincott Williams & Wilkins.

2. Bennett, D. H. (2002) *Cardiac Arrhythmias: Practical Notes on Interpretation and Treatment*, 6th edn, London, Arnold.
3. Beverage, D., Haworth, K., Labus, D., Mayer, B. and Munson, S. (2005) *ECG Interpretation Made Incredibly Easy*, London, Lippincott Williams & Wilkins.
4. Braunwald, E., Zipes, D. and Libby, P. (2001) *Heart Disease: A Textbook of Cardiovascular Medicine*, 6th edn, Philadelphia, PA, W.B. Saunders Co.
5. Fetzer, S. J. (2003) 'The patient with an implantable cardioverter defibrillator', *Journal of Peri-Anesthesia Nursing*, **18**(6): 398–405.
6. Morton, P. G., Fontaine, D. K., Hudak, C. M. and Gallo, B. M. (2005) *Critical Care Nursing: A Holistic Approach*, 8th edn, Philadelphia, PA, Lippincott Williams & Wilkins.
7. Swanton, R. H. (2003) *Cardiology*, 5th edn, Swanton, RH, Blackwell Publishing.
8. Thorn, M. (2006) 'Chest drains: A practical guide', *British Journal of Cardiac Nursing*, **1**(4): 180–5.
9. Van Riper, S. and Van Riper, J. (1997) *Cardiac Diagnostic Tests: A Guide for Nurses*, Philadelphia, PA, W.B. Saunders Co.
10. Wood, M. A. and Ellenbogen, K. A. (2002) 'Cardiac pacemakers from the patient's perspective', *Circulation*, **105**: 1136–8.
11. Woods, S., Froelicher, E. and Motzer, S. (2000) *Cardiac Nursing*, 4th edn, Philadelphia, PA, Lippincott Williams & Wilkins.
12. Yeo, T. P. (2004) 'Counselling patients with implanted cardiac devices', *The Nurse Practitioner*, **29**(12): 58–65.

Glossary of Terms

Aberrant conduction Abnormal pathway of an impulse travelling through the heart's conduction system (1)

Ablate To remove by cutting, erosion, melting, evaporation or vaporisation (6)

Ablation Surgical or radio-frequency removal of an irritable focus in the heart; used to prevent tachyarrhythmias (1)

Accessory pathway A pathway that connects atrial muscle to ventricular muscle or to the lower part of the conduction system and allows either antegrade or retrograde impulse conduction (11)

Acute Having rapid onset, severe symptoms and a short course; not chronic (10)

Aetiology The science that deals with the causation of diseases and their modes of introduction into the host (2)

After load Resistance that the left ventricle must work against to pump blood through the aorta (1)

Akinetic Without movement; in cardiology, usually refers to part of the ventricular wall that is not moving as would be expected (11)

Amplitude Height of a waveform (1)

Anaemia Condition of the blood in which the number of functional red blood cells or the haemoglobin content is below normal (10)

Aneurysm A sac-like enlargement of a blood vessel caused by a weakening of its wall (10)

Angina pectoris A pain in the chest related to reduced coronary circulation due to coronary artery disease or spasms of vascular smooth muscle in coronary arteries (10)

Anterior Nearer to or at the front of the body (10)

Anticoagulant A substance that is able to delay, suppress or prevent the clotting of blood (10)

Anuretic Failure to excrete urine; it may be due to lack of secretion or obstruction in the urinary passages (2)

Aorta The main systemic trunk of the arterial system of the body that emerges from the left ventricle (10)

Apex The pointed end of a conical structure, such as the apex of the heart (10)

Arrhythmia Disturbance of the normal cardiac rhythm from the abnormal origin, discharge or conduction of electrical impulses (1); also called a **dysrhythmia** (10)

Arteriole A small, almost microscopic artery that delivers blood to a capillary (10)

Arteriotomy The surgical opening of an artery (2)

Artery A blood vessel that carries blood away from the heart (10)

Artifact In electrocardiography, any wave or mark on the electrocardiograph that does not represent part of the cardiac cycle. It can be caused by patient movement, poorly placed electrodes or poorly functioning equipment (2)

Ascites Abnormal accumulation of serous fluid in the peritoneal cavity (10)

Asynchronous (fixed-rate) pacing The pacemaker releases a pacing stimulus at the programmed rate, regardless of the heart's intrinsic activity; no sensing occurs, so the pacemaker fires in competition with the heart's natural rhythm; examples of asynchronous modes are AOO, VOO, DOO (12)

Atherosclerosis A process in which fatty substances (cholesterol and triglycerides) are deposited in the walls of medium and large arteries in response to certain stimuli (hypertension, carbon monoxide, dietary cholesterol); following endothelial damage, monocytes stick to the tunica interna, develop macrophages and take up cholesterol and low-density lipoproteins; smooth muscle fibres (cells) in the tunica media ingest cholesterol; this results in the formation of an atherosclerotic plaque that decrease the size of the arterial lumen (9)

Atherosclerotic plaque A lesion that results from accumulated cholesterol and smooth muscle fibres (cells) of the tunica media of the artery; may become obstructive (10)

Atrial fibrillation Asynchronous contraction of the atria that results in the cessation of atrial pumping (10)

Atrial kick Amount of blood pumped into the ventricles as a result of atrial contraction; contributes approximately 30% of total cardiac output (1)

Atrioventricular bundle The part of the conduction system of the heart that begins at the atrioventricular (AV) node, passes through the cardiac skeleton, separating the atria and the ventricles, then runs a short distance down the interventricular septum before splitting into right and left bundle branches; also called the **bundle of His** (10)

Atrioventricular (AV) node The portion of the conduction system of the heart made up of a compact mass of conduction cells located near the orifice of the coronary sinus in the right atrial wall (10)

Atrioventricular (AV) valve A structure made up of membranous flaps or cusps that allow blood flow in one direction only, from an atrium into a ventricle (10)

Atrium A superior chamber of the heart (10)

Auscultation A method of examining internal organs by listening to the sounds they produce (2)

Automaticity Ability of a cardiac cell to initiate an impulse on its own (1)

Base rate The rate at which the pacemaker paces when no intrinsic cardiac activity is present; also called the **minimum rate** or **lower rate** (12)

Benign Innocent, mild, favourable for recovery (2)

Bicuspid valve Atrioventricular valve on the left side of the heart; also called the **mitral valve** (10)

Bipolar Having two poles (1) a pacing lead with two electrical poles; the negative pole is the distal tip of the lead and the positive pole is a metal ring located a few millimetres proximal to the distal tip; the stimulating pulse is delivered through the distal tip electrode; (2) a pacing system with both electrical poles in or on the heart (12)

Blood The fluid that circulates through the heart, arteries, capillaries and veins and that constitutes the chief means of transport within the body (10)

Blood pressure Pressure exerted by blood as it presses against and attempts to stretch blood vessels, especially arteries; the force is generated by the rate and force of heartbeat; clinically, a measure of the pressure in arteries during ventricular systole and ventricular diastole (10)

Bradycardia A slow resting heart or pulse rate (under 50 bpm) (10)

Bruce Protocol Procedures for cardiac stress tests in which the patients gradually increase exercise intensity; used with the exercise portion of nuclear medicine tests (11)

Brugada Syndrome A very rare condition in which the right bundle branch block is accompanied by ST elevation in leads V2 and V3; it is associated with serious ventricular arrhythmias and sudden cardiac death (5)

Bruit An extra whooshing sound heard on auscultation over a blood vessel, gland or organ; when heard over an artery, it is produced by the passage of blood over an irregular surface or through a narrowed portion of the vessel; it may indicate the presence of an aneurysm (2)

Bundle branch block Slowing or blocking of an impulse as it travels through one of the bundle branches (1)

Capillary A microscopic blood vessel located between the arteriole and venule through which materials are exchanged between blood and interstitial fluid (10)

Capture Ability of the pacing stimulus to depolarise the chamber being paced; capture is recognised on the electrocardiogram whenever the pacing spike is followed immediately by the appropriate waveform: an atrial spike followed by a *P* wave or a ventricular spike followed by a wide QRS (12)

Cardiac arrest Cessation of an effective heartbeat in which the heart is completely stopped or in ventricular fibrillation (10)

Cardiac catheterisation An invasive procedure in which a long, flexible radio-opaque catheter is introduced to the heart via the arterial or venous system to visualise the heart's chambers, valves and blood vessels; it may also be used to measure pressure, assess left-ventricular function and cardiac output; to identify the location of septal and valvular defects; and to take tissue and blood samples (10)

Cardiac cycle A complete heartbeat consisting of systole (contraction) and diastole (relaxation) of both atria plus systole and diastole of both ventricles (10)

Cardiac muscle Striated muscle fibres (cells) that form the wall of the heart; stimulated by an intrinsic conduction system and autonomic motor neurons (10)

Cardiac output Amount of blood ejected from the left ventricle per minute; normal value is 4–8 l/minute (10)

Cardiac tamponade Compression of the heart due to excessive fluid or blood in the pericardial sac that could result in heart failure (10)

Cardiomegaly Heart enlargement (10)

Cardiology The study of the heart and the diseases associated with it (10)

Cardiomyopathy A progressive disorder in which ventricular structure or function is impaired; in dilated cardiomyopathy, the ventricles enlarge (stretch) and become weaker and reduce the heart's pumping action; in hypertrophy cardiomyopathy, the ventricular wall thickens and the pumping efficiency of the ventricles is reduced (10)

Cardioversion Restoration of normal rhythm by electric shock or drug therapy (1)

Cardioverter An instrument used to deliver a brief direct-current electric shock to the heart to terminate certain arrhythmias (2)

Carotid sinus massage Manual pressure applied to the carotid sinus to slow the heart rate (1)

Catheter A tube that can be inserted into a body cavity through a canal or into a blood vessel; used to remove fluids, such as urine or blood, and to introduce diagnostic material and medication (9)

Cerebrovascular accident (CVA) Destruction of brain tissue (infarction) resulting from obstruction or rupture of blood vessels that supply the brain; also called **stroke** (10)

Cholesterol Classified as a lipid, the most abundant steroid in animal tissues; located in cell membranes and used for the synthesis of steroid hormones and bile salts (10)

Chordae tendinae Fine, white, glistening cords, stretching between the atrioventricular valves and the papillary muscles of the heart; when the muscles contract, the chordae are tightened, thus preventing the cusps of the atrioventricular valves from being swept back into the atria during ventricular contraction (2)

Chronic Long-term or frequently recurring; applied to a disease that is not acute (10)

Chronographic Having an effect on the rate of rhythmic movement, e.g. the heartbeat (2)

Circus re-entry Delayed impulse in a one-way conduction path in which the impulse remains active and re-enters the surrounding tissues to produce another impulse (1)

Clot The end result of a series of biochemical reactions that changes liquid plasma into a gelatinous mass; specifically, the conversion of fibrinogen into a tangle of polymerised fibrin molecules (10)

Coagulation Process by which a blood clot is formed (10)

Coarctation of the aorta A pressing together or narrowing of the aorta or part of it; may be a congenital heart defect or may be due to pathological narrowing of the median coat of the artery (2)

Commissure The point or line between two parts, e.g. the connecting point of the valve leaflets in the mitral valve (2)

Compensatory pause Period following a premature contraction during which the heart regulates itself, allowing the sinoatrial node to resume normal conduction (1)

Computed tomography (CT) The taking of repeated x-ray slices at multiple angles around a section of the body; the resulting transverse section of the body called a CT scan is reproduced on a video monitor; this procedure visualises soft tissues and organs with much more detail than conventional radiographs; differing tissue densities show up as various shades of grey; multiple scans can be assembled to build three-dimensional views of structures (10); this was previously referred to as a CAT scan (computerised axial tomography) (11)

Conduction Transmission of electrical impulses through the myocardium (1)

Conduction system A group of autorhythmic cardiac muscle fibres that generates and distributes electrical impulses to stimulate coordinated contraction of the heart chambers: including the SA node, the AV node, the AV bundle, the right and left bundle and the Purkinje fibres (10)

Conductivity Ability of one cardiac cell to transmit an electrical impulse to another cell (1)

Contractility Ability of a cardiac cell to contract after receiving an impulse (1)

Contrast A material opaque to x-rays that is given intravenously to increase the difference on an x-ray image between vascular structures (where the contrast is more concentrated) and adjoining tissue; may have iodine (iodinated), may not (no iodinated) (11)

Coronary angiogram An invasive procedure in which a radio-opaque catheter is inserted into the openings of the coronary artery under fluoroscopy; radio-opaque contrast dye is injected into the coronary arteries to visualise them (10)

Coronary angioplasty Use of a balloon-tipped catheter to compress atherosclerotic plaque against the wall of a coronary artery, thus opening a stenotic artery and restoring blood flow to affected myocardium (11)

Coronary artery bypass graft (CABG) Surgical procedure in which a portion of a blood vessel is removed from another part of the body and grafted onto a coronary artery so as to bypass an obstruction in the coronary artery; a piece of the grafted blood vessel is sutured between the aorta and the unblocked portion of the coronary artery (10)

Coronary artery disease (CAD) A condition such as atherosclerosis that causes narrowing of coronary arteries so that blood flow to the heart is reduced; the result is **coronary heart disease (CHD)**; any pathological condition that affects the arteries of the heart, particularly those that lessen the flow of the oxygen and other nutrients to the heart muscle; atherosclerosis is the most common cause of CAD, and angina the most important symptom; causes include cigarette smoking, hypertension, diets high in cholesterol, fats, salt and coffee, and deficiency in certain vitamins (2)

Coronary artery spasm A condition in which the smooth muscle of a coronary artery undergoes a sudden contraction, resulting in vasoconstriction (9)

Coronary circulation The pathway followed by the blood from the ascending aorta through the blood vessels supplying the heart and returning to the right atrium; also called **cardiac circulation** (10)

Coronary heart disease (CHD) The heart muscle receives inadequate blood due to an interruption of its blood supply (10)

Coronary occlusion The term used to describe occlusion of the coronary artery by any cause; this may or may not cause myocardial infarction (5)

Coronary sinus A wide venous channel on the posterior surface of the heart that collects the blood from the coronary circulation and returns it to the right atrium (10)

Coronary thrombosis Refers to occlusion of a coronary artery by a thrombus; this may or may not lead to myocardial infarction (5)

Crosstalk The sensing of a signal in one chamber by the sensing circuit in the other chamber, usually used in reference to the sensing of the atrial output pulse by the ventricular channel; crosstalk due to sensing of atrial signals by the ventricular channel causes inhibition of ventricular pacing output because the ventricular channel interprets the atrial output as a ventricular event (12)

Cutaneous Pertaining to the skin (10)

Defibrillation The arrest of fibrillation of the cardiac muscle (atrial or ventricular) and restoration of normal rhythm; usually refers to treatment by application of electric shock (2)

Defibrillation threshold (DFT) Can be defined as the minimal energy that terminates ventricular fibrillation (3)

Deflection Direction of a waveform, based on the direction of a current (1)

Demand pacing The pacemaker paces only when the heart's intrinsic rate is below the pacemaker's programmed rate, that is only paces when the heart is too slow (7)

Depolarisation Response of a myocardial cell to an electrical impulse that causes movement of ions across the cell membrane, which triggers myocardial contraction (1)

Diabetes insipidus A condition caused by defects in anti-diuretic hormone (ADH) receptors or an inability to secrete ADH and characterised by excretion of large amounts of urine and thirst (10)

Diabetes mellitus A condition caused by an inability to produce or use insulin and characterised by hyperglycemia, increased urine production, excessive thirst and excessive eating (10)

Diaphoresis Perspiration, particularly that which is excessive (2)

Diastole Phase of the cardiac cycle when both atria (atrial diastole) or both ventricles (ventricular diastole) are at rest and filling with blood (1)

Diastolic blood pressure The force exerted by blood on arterial walls during ventricular relaxation; the lowest blood pressure measured in the large arteries (10)

Diathermy The passage of a high-frequency electric current through tissue where heat is produced; it can be used in surgery to stop bleeding (2)

Diathesis An inherited predisposition or combination of attributes that makes a person susceptible to certain diseases or class of diseases (2)

Dissection The act of separating tissue (2)

Distal Farthest from the head, centre or any point of reference; located away from the centre of the body and towards the extremities (2)

Diuresis Increased secretion and excretion of urine (2)

Dizziness A disturbed, unpleasant sense of one's relationship to space, in which objects seem to whirl about; giddiness; may be due to disturbance in any of the body systems that normally keep a person aware of his or her position in space (2)

Dual chamber pacing Pacing in both the atria and ventricles to restore artificially atrioventricular synchrony (7)

Dyskinetic With inappropriate movement; in cardiology, refers to an area of ventricular wall that moves in the opposite direction of normal (such as outward) during systole (11)

Dysplasia Abnormal development of organs, tissues or cells (2)

Dyspnoea Shortness of breath; painful or laboured breathing (10)

ECG complex Waveform representing electrical events of one cardiac cycle; consists of five main waveforms (labelled P, Q, R, S and T), a sixth waveform (labelled *U*) that occurs under certain conditions, the PR and QT intervals, and the ST segment (1)

Echocardiogram A procedure that uses ultrasound waves to obtain an image of the interior of the heart (10)

Ectopic Refers to an impulse arising from any focus other than the sinus node (11)

Ectopic beat Contraction that occurs as a result of an impulse generated from a site other than the sinoatrial node (1)

Elasticity The ability of tissue to return to original shape after contraction or extension (10)

Electrocardiogram (ECG or EKG) A recording of the electrical changes that accompany the cardiac cycle and can be recorded on the surface of the body; may be resting, stress or ambulatory (10)

Electrode The exposed metal tip of a pacing lead that contacts myocardium and directly transmits the pacing stimulus to cardiac tissue (12)

Electromagnetic interference Electrical signals from the environment (i.e. radio-frequency waves) that can be sensed by the pacemaker and interfere with pacer function; abbreviated **EMI** (12)

Embolism Obstruction or closure of a vessel by a piece of foreign matter such as an embolus (2)

Embolus A blood clot, bubble of air, fat from broken bones, mass of bacteria or other debris or foreign material transported by the blood (10)

Empyema A collection of pus in the pleural cavity (8)

Encapsulated Surrounded by a gelatinous or membranous capsule (6)

Enhanced automaticity Condition in which pacemaker cells increase the firing rate above their inherent rate (1)

Epicardium The thin outer layer of the heart wall, composed of serous tissue and mesothelium; also called the **visceral pericardium** (10)

Erythema Skin redness usually caused by dilation of the capillaries (10)

Escape interval The period between a sensed cardiac event and the next pacemaker output; the escape interval is usually equal to the basic pacing rate, but it can be programmed longer in some pacemakers (hysteresis) (12)

Excitability Ability of a cardiac cell to respond to an electrical stimulus (1)

Excretion The process of eliminating waste products from a cell, tissue or the entire body; or the products excreted (12)

Extrinsic Not inherently part of the cardiac electrical system (1)

Fistula An abnormal passage between two organs or between an organ cavity and the outside (10)

Fluoroscope A device for immediate projection of an x-ray image on a fluorescent screen for visual examination of the deeper structures of the body (2)

Fluoroscopy A radiographic technique used to examine a part of the body that allows for immediate serial images (11)

Fossa ovalis cordis A depression on the right side of the interarterial septum of the heart; it represents the remains of the fetal foramen ovale (2)

Fusion beat A cardiac depolarisation (either atrial or ventricular) that results from two foci, both contributing to depolarisation of the chamber; in pacing, a fusion beat results when an intrinsic depolarisation and a pacing stimulus occur simultaneously and both contribute to depolarisation (usually seen in the ventricle) (12)

Graft Tissue or organ transplanted to another part of the body (2)

Groin The depression between the thigh and the trunk; the inguinal region (10)

Group 1 drivers Include motor cars and motorcycles (4)

Group 2 drivers Include large lorries (category C) and buses (category D); the medical standards are much higher than those of group 1 because of the size and weight of the vehicle and also the length of time the driver may spend at the wheel in the course of his/her occupation (4)

Haematoma A tumour or swelling filled with blood (9)

Haemoglobin A substance in erythrocytes (red blood cells) consisting of the protein globin and the iron-containing red pigment heme that transports most of the oxygen and carbon dioxide in the blood (10)

Haemorrhage Bleeding; the escape of blood from vessels, especially when it is profuse (10)

Haemostasis The stoppage of bleeding (10)

Haemostat An agent or instrument used to prevent the flow or escape of blood (9)

Haemothorax The presence of bloody fluid in the pleural cavity (2)

Heart A hollow muscular organ lying slightly to the left of the midline of the chest that pumps the blood through the cardiovascular system (10)

Heart block An arrhythmia (dysrhythmia) of the heart in which the atria and ventricles contract independently because of a blocking of electrical impulses through the heart at some point in the conduction system (10)

Heartburn Burning sensation in the oesophagus due to reflux of hydrochloric acid (HCl) from the stomach (10)

Heart murmur An abnormal sound that consists of a flow noise that is heard before the normal lubb-dupp or that may mask normal heart sounds (10)

Hematocrit (Hct) The percentage of blood made up of red blood cells; usually measured by centrifuging a blood sample in a graduated tube and then reading off the volume of red blood cells and dividing it by the volume of blood in the sample (10)

Holter monitor Electrocardiograph worn by a person while going about everyday routines (9)

Hyperglycaemia An elevated blood sugar level (10)

Hyperkalaemia An above-normal concentration of potassium in blood (10)

Hypertension High blood pressure (10)

Hypertrophic cardiomyopathy Hypertrophy refers to an increase in the bulk of a tissue or structure; cardiomyopathy refers to a disorder of the heart muscle; therefore, hypertrophic cardiomyopathy refers to the enlargement of the ventricles in the absence of any obvious cause (2)

Hypertrophy An excessive enlargement or overgrowth of tissue without cell division (10)

Hypoglycaemia An abnormally low concentration of glucose in the blood; can result from excess insulin (injected or secreted) (10)

Hypokalaemia Deficiency of potassium in the blood (10)

Hypokinetic Having diminished movement; in cardiology, refers to a ventricular wall that is moving less vigorously than normal (11)

Hypotension A blood pressure of less than 90 mmHg or a reduction of greater than 40 mmHg from the patient's baseline (7)

Hypovolaemic shock A type of shock characterised by decreased intravascular volume resulting from blood loss; may be caused by acute haemorrhage or excessive fluid loss (10)

Hysteresis A programmable feature in some pacemakers that allows the escape interval to be programmed longer than the basic pacing interval (the pacing interval after a sensed beat is longer than the basic pacing interval); this allows more time for the heart's intrinsic activity to occur (12)

Iatrogenic The inadvertent development of a secondary illness or condition through medical or surgical treatment for a primary disorder (2)

Idiosyncratic reaction A reaction that is completely different from the one expected; usually refers to drugs which may produce a reaction that is completely opposite to the one which the drug was expected to produce (2)

Imaging In nuclear medicine, composition of a picture by use of a gamma-ray counter, or scintillation camera, which detects and localises the radioactive tracer in the body (11)

Implantation The insertion of a tissue or a part into the body (10)

Infarction The presence of a localised area of necrotic tissue, produced by inadequate oxygenation of the tissue (10)

Infection Invasion and multiplication of micro-organisms in body tissues (10)

Inferior Away from the head or toward the lower part of the structure (10)

Inferior vena cava Large vein that collects blood from parts of the body inferior to the heart and returns it to the right atrium (10)

Inguinal Pertaining to the groin (10)

Inhibited response A type of response to sensing that inhibits pacemaker output when an intrinsic beat is sensed; this results in demand pacing, or pacing only when the heart's intrinsic activity is slower than the basic pacing rate (12)

Inspiration The act of drawing air into the lungs (9)

Insulin A hormone produced by the beta cells of the pancreas that decreases the blood glucose level (10)

Intima Innermost lining of the artery (11)

Intrinsic Naturally occurring electrical stimulus from within the heart's conduction system (1)

Ischaemia A transient and reversible insult to the myocardium as a result of insufficient oxygen supply to the heart tissue (11)

Isoelectric line The baseline of the ECG from which all wave measurements begin and end (11)

Keloid An overgrowth of scar tissue, consisting of a shiny, firm, usually elevated, benign, thickened mass of fibrous tissue forming at the site of a burn, skin wound or surgical incision; may produce a constriction deformity (2)

Late electrical potentials Cardiac electrical activity that occurs after depolarisation; predisposes the patient to ventricular tachycardia (1)

Lead The insulated wire and its electrode that transmits the pacing stimuli from the pulse generator to the heart and relays sensed intrinsic activity back to the pulse generator; a single-chamber pacemaker uses one lead and a dual-chamber pacemaker uses two leads: one in the atrium and one in the ventricle (7)

Lithotripsy The operation of crushing a stone in the urinary bladder and removing the fragments by irrigation (2)

Long QT syndrome A prolonged QT interval during the ventricular depolarisation–repolarisation cycle; increases the risk of ventricular tachycardia (1)

Lumen The space within an artery, vein, intestine or a tube (10)

Magnet mode The pacemaker's response when a magnet is placed over the pulse generator; a magnet inactivates the sensing circuitry and causes a pacemaker to function asynchronously at a predetermined rate and in a pre-set manner; the magnet mode differs among manufacturers in pacing rate and number of impulses delivered with the magnet in place; a change in magnet-induced pacing rate is often an indicator of battery depletion and warrants pulse generator replacement (12)

Magnetic resonance imaging (MRI) During the procedure, the body is exposed to a high-energy magnetic field, which causes the protons (small positive particles within atoms, such as hydrogen) in body fluids and tissues to arrange themselves in relation to the field; then, a pulse radio wave 'reads' these ion patterns, and a colour-coded image is assembled on a video monitor; the result is a two or three-dimensional blueprint of cellular chemistry; the MRI shows fine detail of soft tissue but not bones; can be used to detect artery clogging fatty plaques; although this is a relatively safe procedure, it cannot be used on patients with metal in their bodies; it was formerly called **nuclear magnetic resonance (NMR)** (10)

Malaise Discomfort, uneasiness and indisposition, often indicative of infection (9)

Medial Nearer the mid-line of the body or a structure (10)

Monomorphic Form of ventricular tachycardia in which the QRS complexes have a uniform appearance from beat to beat (1)

Multiform or multifocal Type of premature ventricular contractions that have differing QRS configurations as a result of their originating from different irritable sites in the ventricle (1)

Myocardial infarction Necrosis of a portion of heart muscle as a result of inadequate blood supply (5); also called a **heart attack** (10)

Nephropathy Any disease of the kidney (2)

Nephrotoxic Toxic or destructive to the cells of the kidney (2)

Non-sustained ventricular tachycardia Ventricular tachycardia that lasts less than 30 seconds (1)

Occlusion The act of closure or state of being closed (9)

Oedema Local or general swelling due to the accumulation of fluids in the cells, intercellular spaces and serous cavities (2)

Oesophagus A hollow muscular tube connecting the pharynx and the stomach (10)

Opacify Injection of contrast dye into the coronary artery so that it is no longer transparent under fluoroscopy (6)

Orifice An entrance or outlet of a vessel (11)

Output The electrical stimulus delivered by the pulse generator, usually defined in terms of pulse amplitude (volts) and pulse width (milliseconds) (12)

Overdrive pacing A method to suppress a tachycardia by pacing the heart at a rate faster than the patient's intrinsic heart rate (7)

Oversensing Detection of inappropriate electrical signals by the pacemaker's sensing circuit, resulting in inappropriate inhibition of the pacemaker output (7)

Pacemaker Group of cells that generates impulses to the heart muscle or a battery-powered device that delivers an electrical stimulus to the heart to cause myocardial depolarisation (1)

Pacemaker syndrome Adverse clinical signs and symptoms due to inadequate timing of atrial and ventricular contraction; the syndrome can be due to loss of atrioventricular (AV) synchrony in VVI pacing, inappropriate AV interval in dual-chamber pacing, or inappropriate rate modulation; symptoms include fatigue, confusion, unpleasant pulsations in neck or chest, limited exercise capacity, congestive heart failure, hypotension, and syncope or near syncope (12)

Pacing interval The time between two consecutive paced events without an intervening sensed event; measured in milliseconds; AA interval = atrial pacing interval, VV interval = ventricular pacing interval (12)

Pacing spike The small vertical 'blip' recorded on the electrocardiogram with every pacemaker output pulse; the presence of a pacing spike indicates that a stimulus was released by the pacemaker (12)

Pacing threshold The minimum electrical stimulation required to initiate atrial or ventricular depolarisation consistently; it is usually measured in milliamps (mA) (7)

Paroxysmal Episode of an arrhythmia that starts and stops suddenly (1)

Patent ductus arteriosus (PDA) The ductus arteriosus is a temporary blood vessel between the aorta and the pulmonary trunk; in some babies, this temporary artery remains open rather than closing shortly after birth; as a result, aortic blood flows into the lower-pressure pulmonary trunk, thus increasing the pulmonary trunk blood pressure and overworking both ventricles; in uncomplicated PDA, medication can be used to facilitate the closure of the defect; in more severe cases, surgical intervention may be required (12)

Percutaneous Refers to the insertion of a catheter into the body through a small puncture in the skin, usually into an artery (3)

Peri Prefix denoting (1) all around about; (2) near; (3) enclosing, surrounding (2)

Pericardial cavity Small potential space between the visceral and parietal layers of the serous pericardium that contains pericardial fluid (10)

Pericardium A loose-fitting membrane that encloses the heart, consisting of an outer fibrous layer and an inner serous layer (10)

Peripheral Located on the outer part or a surface of the body (10)

Plaque A layer of dense proteins on the inside of a plasma membrane; a mass of bacterial cells, dextran (polysaccharide) and the other debris that adheres to teeth (10)

Plasma The extra-cellular fluid found in blood vessels; blood minus the formed elements (10)

Platelet plug Aggregation of platelets (thrombocytes) at a site where a blood vessel is damaged that helps to stop or slow blood loss (10)

Plethora fullness; overloading; used especially to describe a condition of overfullness of the blood vessels accompanied by congestion of tissue (2)

Pneumothorax Air or gas in the pleural cavity; causes severe pain, dyspnoea, absence of breath sounds, abnormal distension of the chest (2)

Positron emission topography (PET) During this procedure, a substance that emits positrons (positively charged particles) is injected into the body, where it is taken up by tissues; the collision of positrons with negatively charged electrons in body tissues produces gamma rays (similar to x-rays) that are detected by gamma cameras positioned around the patient; a computer receives signals for the gamma cameras and constructs a PET scan image and displays it in colour on a video monitor; the PET scan shows where the injected substance is being used in the body (10)

Posterior Nearer to or at the back of the body; also called **dorsal** (10)

Pre-excitation Activation of part of the ventricular myocardium earlier than would be expected if the activating impulses travelled only along the normal pathways (11)

Preload Stretching force exerted on the ventricular muscle by the blood that it contains at the end of diastole (1)

Pro-arrhythmia Rhythm disturbance caused or made worse by drugs or other therapy (1)

Prophylactic Acting to defend against, or prevent something, particularly infection or disease (2)

Pseudofusion beat An electrocardiographic phenomenon resulting from delivery of a pacemaker spike into an intrinsic event; in the ventricle, it appears as a pacing spike in an intrinsic QRS complex, but because the ventricle is already depolarised, the spike is ineffective but may distort the QRS complex on the electrocardiogram (12)

Pulmonary embolism The presence of a blood clot or other foreign substance in a pulmonary arterial blood vessel that obstructs circulation to lung tissue (12)

Pulsatile Beating, throbbing (2)

Pulse generator The device that contains the power source (battery) and the electronic circuits that control the artificial pacemaker function; the term 'pacemaker' is commonly used for the pulse generator (7)

QRS wave The deflection wave of an electrocardiogram that represents onset of ventricular depolarisation (10)

Radio frequency (RF) Electromagnetic energy in the megahertz (radio) band of the spectrum; used in MRI to energise hydrogen nuclei, which re-emit the RF energy, forming the MR image (11)

Radio-nuclide scanning During the procedure, a radio nuclide (radioactive substance) is introduced intravenously into the body and carried by the blood to the tissue to be imaged; gamma rays emitted by the radio nuclide are detected by gamma cameras positioned around the patient; a computer receives signals from the gamma cameras and constructs a radio nuclide image and displays it in colour on a video monitor; areas of intense colour take up a lot of radionuclide and represent high tissue activity; areas of less intense colour take up smaller amounts of the radionuclide and represent low tissue activity (10)

Rate modulation The ability of a pacemaker to increase the pacing rate in response to physical activity or metabolic demand the pacemaker uses some type of physiologic sensor to determine the need for increased pacing rate; the most commonly used sensors are motion sensors and minute ventilation sensors; also called rate adaptation or rate response (12)

Redistribution On thallium scans, the process by which thallium will only slowly fill in an ischaemic area of myocardium; thus, on initial (exercise) scan, the area takes up little or no thallium; over time, however, as thallium continues to move from the bloodstream into tissue, the area will show an increase in thallium level; when a two-part thallium scan shows redistribution, this indicates ischaemia; also called **reversible defects** (11)

Re-entry mechanism Failure of a cardiac impulse to follow the normal conduction pathway; instead, it follows a circular path (1)

Refractory period (1) In the heart, the period of time for which the myocardium is incapable of responding to a stimulus; (2) In the pacemaker, an interval or timing cycle following a sensed or paced event during which the pacemaker does not respond to incoming signals; a single-chamber pacemaker has one refractory period, and a dual-chamber pacemaker has an atrial refractory and a ventricular refractory period (12)

Repolarisation Recovery of the myocardial cells after depolarisation during which the cell membrane returns to its resting potential (1)

Revascularisation Restoration of blood supply to an affected area of myocardium, such as by angioplasty or thrombolytic therapy (11)

Rhythm strip Length of ECG paper that shows multiple ECG complexes representing a picture of the heart's electrical activity in a specific lead (1)

Sensing The ability of the pacemaker to recognise and respond to intrinsic cardiac depolarisation (12)

Sensing threshold The smallest intrinsic atrial or ventricular signal (measured in millivolts) that can be consistently sensed by the pacemaker (12)

Sensitivity The relative ability of a test to detect the desired disease entity when that condition is present; for instance, when a test has a sensitivity of 90%, the test will be positive for 90% of those who have the disease (12)

Sequela An after-effect of disease, injury or surgery (6)

Seroma An accumulation of serum usually under the skin, which produces a swelling resembling a tumour (2)

Shock Failure of the cardiovascular system to deliver adequate amounts of oxygen and nutrients to meet the metabolic needs of the body due to inadequate cardiac output; it is characterised by hypotension, clammy, cool and pale skin, sweating, reduced urine formation, altered mental state, acidosis, tachycardia, weak and rapid pulse, and thirst; types include hypovolaemic, carcinogenic, vascular and obstructive (10)

Shunt A pathway through which blood flows in an unusual or abnormal direction (11)

Silent ischaemia Ischaemia in the absence of symptoms; the term is applied particularly to episodes of ST elevation or depression unaccompanied by pain (5)

Single-photon emission computerised topography (SPECT) Nuclear-imaging technique in which many scans are taken as slices of the subject by a moving camera and reassembled by computer into a detailed composite picture of the patient (11)

Slice In CT and MRI scanning, the thin x-ray cut that produces a cross-sectional image; likened to slicing a cucumber and viewing it end-on (11)

Stenosis Narrowing or closure of a blood vessel due to the build up of plaque on the intimal surface (11)

Stimulation threshold The minimum amount of voltage necessary to capture the heart consistently; also called capture threshold or pacing threshold (12)

Stokes–Adams attack Sudden episode of light-headedness or loss of consciousness caused by an abrupt slowing or stopping of the heartbeat (1)

Stroke volume The amount of blood ejected by the left ventricle at each heartbeat (2)

Superior Toward the head or upper part of a structure (10)

Superior vena cava Large vein that collects blood from the body superior to the heart and returns it to the right atrium (10)

Supraventricular Originating at or above the atrioventricular junction (11)

Sustained ventricular tachycardia Type of ventricular tachycardia that lasts longer than 30 seconds (1)

Sympathomimetic Capable of producing changes similar to those produced by stimulation of the sympathetic nerves (2)

Syncope A transient loss of consciousness followed by spontaneous recovery (11)

Systole Phase of the cardiac cycle in which both of the atria (atrial systole) or the ventricles (ventricular systole) are contracting (1)

Tachyarrhythmia A heartbeat of 100 or more per minute; it may or may not be regular (1; 10)

Tamponade Pathological compression of an organ as in cardiac tamponade (2)

Tetralogy of Fallot A combination of four congenital heart defects: (1) constricted pulmonary semilunar valve; (2) interventricular septal opening; (3) emergence of aorta from both ventricles instead of from the left only; and (4) enlarged right ventricle (10)

Thermodilution A technique of measuring the cardiac output during right-sided catheterisation; using the Swan–Ganz catheter, which has two separate lumens: one opening into the right atrium and the other into the pulmonary artery; this technique is based on the principle that the concentration of an injected substance is dependent on the volume injected and the volume of blood into which it is injected via the catheter into the right atrium; the temperature is then sampled on the pulmonary artery as the cold saline, diluted in the blood, passes the thermistor at the catheter tip; the transient fall in blood temperature is, therefore, indirectly related to the cardiac output, that is the greater the fall in temperature, the lower the cardiac output for a given volume of saline injected (5)

Thigh The portion of the lower extremity between the hip and the knee (10)

Thorax The chest (10)

Thrombin The active enzyme formed from prothrombin that acts to convert fibrinogen to fibrin (10)

Thrombolytic drugs Pharmacologic agents (e.g. streptokinase, tissue plasminogen activator (t-PA) and urokinase) used to dissolve blood clots, particularly in the setting of acute MI (11)

Thrombophlebitis A disorder in which inflammation of the wall of a vein is followed by the formation of a blood clot (thrombus) (9)

Thrombosis The formation of a clot in an unbroken blood vessel, usually in a vein (10)

Thrombus A clot formed in an unbroken vessel, usually a vein (10)

Thyrotoxicosis A condition due to excessive production of the thyroid gland hormone, thyroxin; signs and symptoms include increased metabolic rate, anxiety, nervousness, tachycardia, sweating, heat intolerance, emotional lability, increased appetite and loss of weight, a fine tremor of the hands when outstretched, and prominence of the eyes (2)

Tine A prong; like a fork (6)

Tissue plasminogen activator (t-PA) An enzyme that dissolves small blood clots by initiating a process that converts plasminogen to plasmin, which degrades the fibrin of a clot (10)

Toxic Pertaining to poison (9)

Transcutaneous Pertaining to the passage of a substance through the unbroken skin (2)

Transfusion Transfer of whole blood, blood components or bone marrow directly into the bloodstream (10)

Trans-septal Across the septum (11)

Tricuspid Atrioventricular (AV) valve on the right side of the heart (10)

Trigeminy Premature beat occurring every third beat that alternates with two normal QRS complexes (1)

Triglyceride A lipid formed from one molecule of glycerol and three molecules of fatty acids that may be either solid (fats) or liquid (oils) at room temperature; the body's most highly concentrated source of chemical potential energy; also called **neutral fat** (10)

Ultrasound Medical imaging technique that utilises high-frequency sound waves to reflect off body tissue to obtain an image of that tissue; the image which may be still or moving is called a **sonogram**; this is a safe, non-invasive, painless procedure that does not use any dye; most commonly used to visualise the fetus during pregnancy (10)

Undersensing Failure of a pacemaker to sense intrinsic cardiac depolarisation; this can result in competition between the pacemaker and the intrinsic rhythm (7)

Uniform or unifocal Type of premature ventricular contraction that has the same or similar QRS configuration and that originates from the same irritable site in the ventricle (1)

Unipolar Having one pole; (1) a unipolar lead has only one pole, located at the distal tip; (2) a pacing system with one pole in or on the heart and the second pole located remote from the heart to complete the circuit; permanent unipolar systems use the back of the pulse generator as the second pole; temporary epicardial pacing systems use a ground wire in subcutaneous tissue as the second pole (12)

Uraemia Accumulation of toxic levels of urea and other nitrogenous waste products in the blood, usually resulting from severe kidney malfunction (10)

Urine The fluid produced by the kidneys that contains wastes and excess materials; excreted from the body through the urethra (10)

Urticaria A skin eruption characterised by circumscribed, smooth, itchy, raised welts that are either redder or paler than the surrounding skin, developing suddenly, usually lasting a few days, and leaving no visible trace (2)

Vagal Pertaining to the vagus nerve (2)

Vagal stimulation Pharmacologic or manual stimulation of the vagus nerve to slow the heart rate (1)

Valsalva's manoeuvre Technique of forceful expiration against a closed glottis; used to slow the heart rate (1)

Varicose Pertaining to an unnatural swelling, as in the case of a varicose vein (10)

Vascular Pertaining to or containing many blood vessels (10)

Vascular spasm Contraction of the smooth muscle in the wall of a damaged blood vessel to prevent blood loss (10)

Vasoconstriction A decrease in the size of the lumen of a blood vessel caused by contraction of the smooth muscle in the wall of the vessel (10)

Vasodilation An increase in the size of the lumen of a blood vessel caused by relaxation of the smooth muscle in the wall of the vessel (10)

Vasovagal reaction Stimulation of the vagus nerve, resulting in a decreased heart rate and decreased blood pressure (11)

Vein A blood vessel that conveys blood from tissues back to the heart (10)

Vena cava One of two large veins that open into the right atrium, returning to the heart all of the deoxygenated blood from the systemic circulation except from coronary circulation (10)

Ventricle A cavity in the brain or an inferior chamber of the heart (10)

Ventricle fibrillation Asynchronous ventricular contractions; unless reversed by defibrillation, results in cardiovascular failure (10)

Venule A small vein that collects blood from capillaries and delivers it to a vein (10)

Vomiting Forcible expulsion of the contents of the upper gastrointestinal tract through the mouth (10)

REFERENCES

1. Beverage, D., Haworth, K., Labus, D., Mayer, B. and Munson, S. (2005) *ECG Interpretation Made Incredibly Easy*, London, Lippincott Williams & Wilkins.
2. *Blackwells Dictionary of Nursing* (1994) London.
3. Braunweld, E., Zipes, D. and Libby, P. (2001) *Heart Disease: A Textbook of Cardiovascular Medicine*, Vol. 1, 6th edn, London, W.B. Saunders Co.
4. DVLA (2006) *For Medical Practitioners: At a Glance Guide to the Current Medical Standards for Fitness to Drive*, February, available online at *www.DVLA.gov.uk.*
5. Julian, D. G., Cowan, J. C. and McLenachan, J. M. (2005) *Cardiology*, 8th edn, London, Elsevier Saunders.
6. *Longman Dictionary of the English Language* (1991).
7. Morton, P. G., Fontaine, D. K., Hudak, C. M. and Gallo, B. M. (2005) *Critical Care Nursing: A Holistic Approach*, 8th edn, Philadelphia, PA, Lippincott Williams & Wilkins.
8. Thorn, M. (2006) 'Chest drains: A practical guide', *British Journal of Cardiac Nursing*, 1(4).
9. Tortora, G. J. and Grabowski, S. R. (1993) *Principles of Anatomy and Physiology*, 7th edn, Menlo Park, CA, Harper Collins College Publishers.
10. Tortora, G. J. and Derrickson, B. (2006) *Principles of Anatomy and Physiology*, 8th edn, Chichester, John Wiley and Sons Inc.
11. Van Riper, S. and Van Riper, J. (1997) *Cardiac Diagnostic Tests: A Guide for Nurses*, London, W.B. Saunders Co.
12. Woods, S., Froelicher, E. and Motzer, S. (2000) *Cardiac Nursing*. 4th edn, Philadelphia, PA, Lippincott Williams & Wilkins.

List of Abbreviations

ACC/AHA	American College of Cardiology/American Heart Association
ACE	Angiotensin-converting enzyme
ACS	Acute coronary syndrome
ACT	Activated clotting time
ADH	Antidiuretic hormone
AF	Atrial fibrillation
AIDS	Acquired immunodeficiency syndrome
AP	Anteroposterior
APD	Action potential duration
APTT	Activated partial thromboplastin time
ARVD	Arrhythmogenic right ventricular dysplasia
AS	Aortic stenosis
ASD	Atrial septal defect
ATP	Anti-tachycardia pacing
AV	Atrioventricular
AVD	Aortic valve disease
AVNRT	Atrioventricular nodal re-entrant tachycardia
AVR	Aortic valve replacement
AVRT	Atrioventricular reciprocating tachycardia
BCIS	British Cardiac Interventional Society
BMS	Bare metal stent
BPEG	British Pacing and Electrophysiology Group
bpm	Beats per minute
CA	Coronary angiogram
CABG	Coronary artery bypass graft surgery
CAD	Coronary artery disease
CCF	Congestive cardiac failure
CCU	Coronary care unit
CHD	Coronary heart disease
CK	Creatine kinase
CK-MB	Creatine kinase myocardial bound
cm	Centimetres
CNS	Central nervous system
CO	Cardiac output
COPD	Chronic obstructive pulmonary disease
CPK-MB	Creatine phosphokinase myocardial bound

CPR	Cardiopulmonary resuscitation
CREDO	Clopidogrel for the Reduction of Events During Observation
CRP	C-reactive protein
CRT	Cardiac resynchronisation therapy
CT	Computed tomography
CURE	Clopidogrel in Unstable Angina to Prevent Recurrent Events
CVA	Cerebrovascular accident
CVP	Central venous pressure
CVS	Cardiovascular system
CXR	Chest x-ray
DC	Direct current
DCA	Directional coronary atherectomy
DCM	Dilated cardiomyopathy
DES	Drug eluting stent
DFP	Diastolic filling period
DFT	Defibrillation threshold
DI	Diabetes insipidus
DVLA	Driver and Vehicle Licensing Agency
ECG	Electrocardiogram
EMI	Electromagnetic interference
EPS	Electrophysiology study
ERI	Elective replacement indicator
ESR	Erythrocyte sedimentation rate
FBC	Full blood count
GFR	Glomerular filtration rate
GP	Glycoprotein
GTN	Glyceryl trinitrate
HCM	Hypertrophic cardiomyopathy
HDL	High-density lipoprotein
HIV	Human immunodeficiency virus
HR	Heart rate
IABP	Intra-aortic balloon pump
ICD	Implantable cardioverter defibrillator
ICS	Intercostal space
ICU	Intensive care unit
IHD	Ischaemic heart disease
IMA	Internal mammary artery
IMPACT	Integrilin to Minimise Platelet Aggregation and Coronary Thrombosis

INR	International normalised ratio
ITU	Intensive therapy unit
IVC	Inferior vena cava
IVUS	Intravascular ultrasound
JVP	Jugular venous pulse
kPa	Kilo pascals
LA	Left atrium
LAD	Left axis deviation/Left anterior descending artery
LAO	Left anterior oblique
LBBB	Left-bundle branch block
LCA	Left coronary artery
LCx	Left circumflex coronary artery
LDH	Lactic dehydrogenase
LDL	Low-density lipoprotein
LFT	Liver function test
LIMA	Left internal mammary artery
LMCA	Left main coronary artery
LMWH	Low-molecular-weight heparin
LPA	Left pulmonary artery
LV	Left ventricle
LVAD	Left ventricular assist device
LVEF	Left ventricular ejection fraction
LVET	Left ventricular ejection time
LVF	Left ventricular fraction
LVH	Left ventricular hypertrophy
MI	Myocardial infarction
ml	Millilitres
mm Hg	Millimetres of mercury
MR	Mitral regurgitation
MRI	Magnetic resonance imaging
MS	Mitral stenosis
MUGA	Multiple-gated acquisition
MV	Mitral valve
mV	Millivolt
MV	Mitral valve
MVR	Mitral valve replacement
NASPE	North American Society of the Pacing and Electrophysiology Group
NMC	Nursing Midwifery Council

NSTEMI   Non-ST-segment elevation myocardial infarction
NYHA   New York Heart Association

PA   Pulmonary artery
PAW   Pulmonary artery wedge
PBMV   Percutaneous balloon mitral valvuloplasty
PCI   Percutaneous coronary intervention
PCV   Packed cell volume
PCW   Pulmonary capillary wedge
PDGF   Platelet-derived growth factor
PES   Programmed electrical stimulation
PET   Positron emission tomography
PFO   Patent foramen ovale
PPM   Permanent pacemaker
PS   Pulmonary stenosis
PTCA   Percutaneous transluminal coronary angioplasty
PUO   Pyrexia of unknown origin
PV   Pulmonary vein

RA   Right atrium
RAD   Right axis deviation
RAO   Right anterior oblique
RBBB   Right-bundle branch block
RCA   Right coronary artery
RF   Radio frequency
RFA   Radio-frequency ablation
RPA   Right pulmonary artery
rpm   Rotations per minute
RV   Right ventricle
RVF   Right ventricular failure
RVH   Right ventricular hypertrophy

SA   Sinoatrial
SR   Sinus rhythm
SSS   Sick sinus syndrome
STEMI   ST-elevation myocardial infarction
SVC   Superior vena cava
SVG   Saphenous vein bypass graft
SVI   Stroke volume index
SVT   Supraventricular tachycardia

TEC   Transluminal extraction catheter
TENS   Transcutaneous electrical nerve stimulation
TGA   Transposition of the great arteries

TIMI	Thrombolysis in myocardial infarction
TNK	Tenecteplase
TOE	Transoesophageal echocardiography
t-PA	Tissue plasminogen activator
TR	Tricuspid regurgitation
TS	Tricuspid stenosis
TSH	Thyroid-stimulating hormone
UA	Unstable angina
UFH	Unfractionated heparin
V	Volts
VF	Ventricular fibrillation
VPB	Ventricular premature beat
VRT	Ventricular resynchronisation therapy
VSD	Ventricular septal defect
VT	Ventricular tachycardia
WBC	White blood cell count
WPW	Wolff–Parkinson–White syndrome

Index